Evidence-based Pharmacy

Regional Pharmaceutical Adviser
NHS, Executive, South East

Co-ordinating Editor
Cochrane Pain, Palliative and Supportive

Radcliffe Medical Press

Radcliffe Medical Press Ltd
18 Marcham Road, Abingdon, Oxon OX14 1AA

British Library Cataloguing in Publication Data

A catalogue record for this book is available from the British Library.

ISBN 1 85775 384 4

Typeset by Acorn Bookwork, Salisbury, Wiltshire
Printed and bound by TJ International Ltd, Padstow, Cornwall

Contents

Preface

The concept for this book came from discussions with Dr Muir Gray, formerly Director of Research and Development at the Anglia & Oxford Region NHSE. Much of the inspiration came from working in the extremely fertile environment of the Oxford Pain Research Unit and *Bandolier* office, headed by Andrew Moore and Henry McQuay. This multidisciplinary unit is a powerhouse of ideas and developments and the best example of a 'can do' culture that I know. Some of the material used in this book has come from *Bandolier*, much has grown out of the work of the Pain Research Unit over recent years and its pioneering work to develop an evidence base for treatments offered to patients suffering pain. Thanks also to Celia Duff and Mike Gill of NHSE for encouragement to publish.

Knowledge of treatment regimens and medicines is constantly changing and every attempt has been made to ensure the accuracy of the data included in this text. Readers are strongly advised to confirm that information, particularly with regard to drug dosage, is accurate and up to date.

The views in this book are those of an individual and do not represent the views of Her Majesty's Government.

Phil Wiffen
May 2001

CHAPTER ONE

Taking pharmacy practice into the 21st century

The practice of pharmacy is once more at a crossroads, as it has been many times before. Opportunities that have been created by both the profession itself and many external pressures threaten old paradigms, but at the same time provide the potential to open up vast opportunities for new areas of practice.

Initiatives such as the Royal Pharmaceutical Society's 'Pharmacy in a New Age' programme encouraged the profession to take a long, hard look at itself and the many issues that impinge on medicine use and pharmacist behaviour. The initiative has given rise to a renewed search for evidence and encouraged the development of a number of related research projects.

The continuing pressure of limited resources will undoubtedly change the way pharmacy is practised. Innovation continues to run ahead of our ability to fund new developments, and demands from an increasingly informed public add to this pressure.

These realities have created a fertile environment for the growth of evidence-based practice. Developments offering to identify effective interventions and providing the possibility of eliminating those activities which are ineffective or even harmful is clearly attractive to many, particularly those who purchase healthcare. There is a further attraction in the dogma that eliminating useless interventions will somehow free up resources for new developments. This is probably wishful thinking. For example, the issue of guidelines on the use of statins for hypercholesterolaemia by the UK Department of Health Standing Medical Advisory Committee (SMAC) in 1997,[1] partly aimed at reducing the growth in use of these drugs, clearly highlighted the underuse of this class of medicines in secondary prevention (seeking to prevent a further myocardial infarction, MI) and is already leading to a steady increase in the use of statins, with an associated increase in expenditure. Such an improvement in care can be shown to provide cost-effective treatment, but it raises issues of affordability. However, other professionals regard the whole evidence-based movement as a threat to their right to practise.

The development of information technology (IT) has greatly facilitated the evidence-based healthcare movement. Bibliographic databases are now accessible from many personal computers (PCs), so that searches can be carried out in the comfort of the office or even at the patient's bedside; the days when this could happen only by appointment with an expert librarian are over. The Internet provides worldwide, almost instant access across continents to good-quality guidelines and protocols for treatment at little cost, informing both professional and patient alike.

Drivers for evidence-based healthcare

Patient expectations

Consumerism has arrived in healthcare, almost certainly aided by the concept of an internal market where money was supposed to follow patients. The age of blindly following doctors' orders is rapidly disappearing and many users are demanding access to services at times that will not interfere with busy work schedules. Day surgery units are increasingly providing evening sessions and private healthcare facilities are offering surgical procedures at a discount during times of lower demand, such as the Christmas break. Patients are becoming increasingly knowledgeable about their conditions. After receiving a diagnosis they may use the Internet both to gain further insight and to identify treatment options, often using the information as a bargaining tool with their clinicians. New developments are featured on prime-time news, on consumer programmes and in popular magazines, leading to an increased demand for the latest and the best treatments as described by the media.

All these developments increase the pressure on healthcare services so that consultations need to be longer to deal with more evidence and the ensuing discussions.

Box 1.1   Three drivers for healthcare demand

- Patient demand
- Population ageing
- Advances in technology

Population ageing

Population ageing is another key factor increasing the demand for healthcare. As the number of older people increases, the demand for healthcare increases simply because old people require more care. Expectations are changing. The generation of elderly people who were mesmerised by the white coat is being replaced with those who have higher expectations and will not settle for poor or inadequate service. An older population will challenge some of our current practices. For example, we will need to offer renal transplants to an older age group than is often the case at present, and insert artificial hips not once but twice. There is already pressure to develop new and effective treatments for some of the diseases of old age such as Alzheimer's disease.

Advances in healthcare technology

In recent years there have been a number of developments targeted at diseases for which, in the past, there was either poor opportunity for treatment or no treatment at all. Procedures that used to require long inpatient stays are now undertaken on a day-case unit. New treatments for schizophrenia have improved the quality of life for many sufferers and there are now treatments emerging for motor neurone disease, multiple sclerosis and Alzheimer's disease. New pharmacological interventions tend to be expensive and some recent developments have not been as effective as had been hoped. It is likely that developments in the pipeline will be increasingly effective and costly.

While the high-cost interventions that benefit relatively small numbers of patients can have a major impact on budgets, equally difficult to manage are the 'medium-cost, medium-volume' developments. Two examples are the use of proton pump inhibitors and statins. The proton pump inhibitor omeprazole became the top-cost drug on all UK health authorities' medicines expenditure in a short space of time and statins are also placing considerable pressure on budgets. Many of these developments can, or have the potential to, save costs elsewhere, such as by reducing the need for hospital admissions, but certainly in the short term the impact is seen as an increased demand for resources.

Professional expectations

The three drivers for healthcare demand described above have an impact on professional expectations. Many professionals want to be at the leading edge in their own fields and are keen to gain experience of the latest developments. An anaesthetist is often keen to gain experience of the latest inhalation anaesthetic, while the oncologist wants to try out the latest chemotherapy. This desire to gain experience of use is not always rational or firmly based on good evidence.

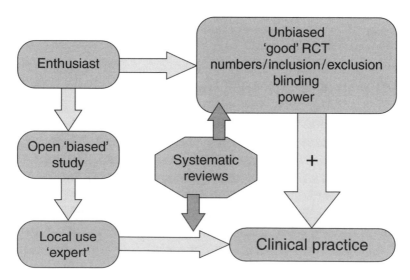

Figure 1.1: How the enthusiast incorporates a new intervention into clinical practice.[2]

Figure 1.1 illustrates what often happens. The enthusiast 'evaluates' a new intervention and quickly becomes the local expert on its use. The intervention is then incorporated into clinical practice, often quite quickly and without the necessary evaluation.

More demanding patients' expectations will inevitably lead to a rise in professional expectations. For example, clinical pharmacists in the course of their rounds are increasingly asked to provide more information on the potentially harmful effects of medication. The depth of answers required often goes beyond a cursory scan of the standard pharmacy reference books or even familiarity with one or two published papers on the subject.

What is the purpose of this book?

Professional practice has to be about doing the right things right. It seeks to answer the questions: How do we know what the right things are? How do we know when we are doing them right? Take the example of blood-level monitoring for a drug with a narrow therapeutic window. We need to know whether blood-level monitoring is of any value, and if it is proven to be of value we need to know when the levels should be measured in the treatment plan and at what time blood should be taken in relation to dosing. Failure to take the blood at the correct time can result in doing the right thing (i.e. monitoring blood levels) wrongly (because the action renders the result meaningless).

Doing the right things

While the objective in healthcare is to do more good than harm, there are many examples of treatment making patients worse than before. Pharmacists are very aware of the need to balance benefit of an improvement with the risk of causing harm either temporarily or permanently. Interventions can have three possible outcomes: (Box 1.2).

Box 1.2   The three possible outcomes for an intervention

- Doing more good than harm
- Doing more harm than good
- Unknown whether of benefit or not

Good implies effective, but it must also be safe and acceptable. Harm is self-evident but is often overlooked in the intensity of treatment. The search for a cure can lead to long-term damage, which may not be reversible. There are many examples of new pharmacological developments where the benefits are actively promoted but the adverse-effect profile only emerges over a considerable period of time. These effects may be caused by the active agent or by additional ingredients or the vehicle used. One example was the use of a polyethoxylated castor oil vehicle for the intravenous anaesthetic agent alphaxalone (Althesin™). This vehicle was later associated with severe anaphylactic reactions, hyperlipidaemias and alterations in blood viscosity.

It is apparent that good and harm have to be weighed for each situation. A toxic treatment may be more acceptable in a life-threatening illness, although patients may not always agree.

Underpinning all this should be an evaluation of the strength of the evidence that informs the evaluation of benefit and risk. As will be shown in Chapter 2, if the expression of good or harm is only based on a personal opinion then it should be discarded. It is important to look for evidence that eliminates the possibility of the result being chance, or of bias.

Table 1.1   Actions needed to improve good

Type of intervention	Action to improve good
Does more good than harm	Promote intervention if affordable
	Seek to improve the good and reduce the harm
Does more harm than good	Prevent the intervention from being introduced
	Stop it if it cannot be improved
Unknown effect	Prevent the intervention from being introduced
	Find out what effect the intervention does have either by systematic review or by appropriate conduct of randomised controlled trials

Table 1.1 outlines the actions that need to be taken when benefit and harm have been assessed.

Strategies to increase the good-to-harm ratio

The time delay from publication to acceptance for a new intervention may be many years. Antman and colleagues compared the results of meta-analyses of randomised controlled trials (RCTs) with clinical expert recommendations for the use of thrombolytic therapy in the treatment of MI in a paper which has become a classic.[3] Figure 1.2 lists the publication dates of the trials, the numbers of published trials and the overall odds ratio showing benefit. The figure shows that by 1975, there was clear evidence of effect. This evidence becomes increasingly stronger as more studies are published.

Even though it was shown that thrombolytic therapy was beneficial in the mid-1970s, these results were not routinely used until

	Cumulative		Odds ratio
Year	RCTs	Patients	
1960	1	23	
	2	65	
	3	149	
1965	4	316	
	7	1793	
1970	10	2544	$p < 0.01$
	11	2651	
1975	15	3311	
	17	3929	
1980	22	5452	
	23	5767	
	27	6125	$p < 0.001$
1985	33	6571	
	65	47185	
1990	70	48154	$p < 0.00001$

Figure 1.2: Results of meta-analyses of RCTs with recommendations for thrombolytic therapy in MI.[3]

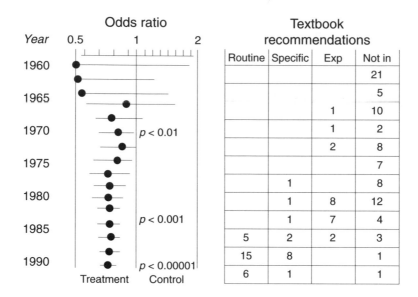

Figure 1.3: Delay in textbook recommendation for thrombolytic therapy in MI.[3]

the late 1980s, a delay of around ten years. The tragedy is that knowledge has not been disseminated or incorporated into the textbooks in a timely fashion. This phenomenon, clearly illustrated by Antman and colleagues, is displayed in Figure 1.3. The key lesson in this is not the indiscriminate use of new interventions but the careful appraisal of evidence and decision making based on this appraisal.

Three battles that pharmacists need to note

Eddy,[4] writing primarily about health reforms in the US, describes three battles that are currently taking place. He argues that the three main goals of healthcare reform are access, quality and cost, but that cost, particularly the rate of increase of cost, is the driving force. The fact that budgets are consistently overspent suggests that healthcare is becoming an uncontrollable item. Eddy further points out that costs will never be controlled unless the decisions made by physicians about treatments, in the widest sense, are challenged and controlled. This will lead to battles over what practitioners do and how they do it. He sees the three battles in this area focusing on evidence, costs and physician autonomy.

Box 1.3   Three battles in healthcare reforms (Eddy)

- Evidence
- Costs
- Physician autonomy

Evidence

Eddy argues that evidence is the first battle, which is made up of three components.

- How much and what type of evidence is sufficient to justify use of a treatment? This covers issues such as what type of evidence is required and how much? If enough experts declare a treatment valuable, is this sufficient?
- The second component surrounds the burden of proof. Should a treatment be considered 'on trial' until there is sufficient proof, or should it be considered effective until proven otherwise?
- The third component is about what we should do with old treatments. The weight of research funding is being applied to new and innovative treatments but there are hundreds of treatments that gained acceptance in the days when the burden of proof required was far less. This may account for 80–90% of available treatments, according to Eddy. Because we do not have the evidence, we do not even know what we do not know.

Costs

The cost of healthcare is a major problem for any government. The battle takes place on several fronts, as we saw with evidence. The most familiar is knowing where to draw the line for the intensity of treatment or for groups of patients. New drug developments in the UK, together with somewhat equivocal supporting evidence, have led to the so-called 'postcode prescribing' phenomenon, where access to treatment largely depends on the health authority catchment area in which a patient happens to reside. For example, patients who live in an area on a health authority border can have different treatments, or even no treatment, depending on which health authority pays the bill. A similar debate is currently taking place over the use of statins. Many would argue that they should be kept for secondary prevention in patients with hyperlipidaemia who have already suffered a MI, but others argue that it is cost-effective to treat hyperlipidaemic patients with a number of risk factors before the MI occurs. If one subscribes to the second argument, then a decision has to be made about the cholesterol level or combination of risk factors that determine whether lipids should be started. There are no easy answers.

The second cost-issue dilemma occurs when there are several treatments for the same problem, and while benefits may differ slightly, the costs differ a great deal. Staying with the statins, some argue that their action is a class effect so it does not matter which statin is used, while others argue that only the more expensive brand leaders should be used because they are supported by large RCT evidence. Somehow, Eddy argues, there has to be a trade-off between quality and cost.

Eddy calls the third area 'It's not much but it's all we've got'. This is where there is only one treatment but the benefits are small even when compared to no treatment. The most difficult examples of this type are the last-hope treatments for cancer. These are the ones that can be very expensive, are extremely emotive, rarely produce benefit and can hit the headlines.

Eddy's fourth point on cost is 'It's all we've got and it is a lot'. He mentions the case of Gaucher's disease, a rare genetic disease (about four cases per million) caused by a deficiency of glucosylceramidase. The results of the disease in children are severe neurological problems and early death. There is now a replacement enzyme available at a cost of between £15 000 and £100 000 per annum, possibly for the rest of a patient's life. A similar argument surrounds the use of total parenteral nutrition for a patient who has undergone a total gastrectomy. While not in the same cost league as Gaucher's disease, the costs involved are a significant sum for any health economy to bear. Remember, money in any budget can only be spent once.

Eddy's final point is on what he calls futile care, treatments that have no reasonable possibility of providing any satisfactory quality of life for the patient. These are almost invariably administered at the wish of a patient's relatives, who want everything possible to be done, or for some sociological argument that it is unacceptable to give up. Eddy reckons that tens of billions of dollars that could be reallocated to provide greater benefit to a wider range of patients are wasted.

It is likely that treatment guidelines to govern some of these scenarios will become increasingly prominent.

Physician autonomy

Eddy's third battle is physician autonomy, which is perceived by many clinicians to be one of the most desirable features of medical practice and is defended by the argument that physicians use their best judgement to provide the best possible care for an individual patient. The battles around evidence and cost challenge this area because judgement may not be evidence-based or even correct, and there may be pressure to get best value for money from limited resources, with the strongest arguments coming from those who are not clinicians. Eddy believes that many practitioners will understand that it is no more insulting to use good-quality guidelines than to obtain advice from a journal. However, pressure may come from both administrators who have an eye on the bottom line and medical colleagues who wish to rein in those who take more than their fair share from the global pot.

Pharmacy practice in the 21st century

Being at the crossroads provides opportunity for indecision or for a decisive shaping of the future. Pharmacy is well-placed to be involved with the management of innovation and knowledge, and there is no reason why pharmacists should not be leading the cultural transformation of the health service by influencing decisions based on current best knowledge of drugs, in terms of both benefits and adverse events.

Pharmacists can add significant value to these processes. However, many of the arguments put forward by Eddy have direct relevance for pharmacists. Clinical pharmacists are already seeking to help clinicians juggle limited resources in secondary care, and physician autonomy has largely disappeared, but pharmacy will need to be sure that its own house is kept in order. For hospital pharmacists the challenge of skill-mix to ensure that pharmacists are put to best use is uppermost, as resources continue to be squeezed. One of the reasons that clinical pharmacy has been able to develop is that technicians have taken over many tasks that pharmacists used to perform.

There is still a need to be constantly evaluating what we do and why we do it, in order to meet the demands of healthcare in the future. There are also new challenges to be faced, such as who the knowledge managers of the future will be. The challenge in community pharmacy is probably greater: the future is likely to belong to those who are willing to develop services, take risks and then seek funding, rather than those with the common attitude of wanting money up front. Current funding mechanisms need to move away from the payment-per-dispensing-item method, greater use will need to be made of technical support and the current practice of having only one pharmacist in each shop almost certainly needs to change.

One thing is sure: whatever is developed will increasingly need to be supported by reliable evidence derived from top-quality research.

References

1   Standing Medical Advisory Committee (1997) The Use of Statins [Web page]. Available at www.open.gov.uk/doh/cmo/statins2.htm

2   Moore A, McQuay H, Gray JAM (1995) Bandolier, *The First 20 Issues*. NHS R&D, Oxford.

3   Antman EM, Lau J, Kupelnick B, Mosteller F, Chalmers TC (1992) A comparison of results of meta-analyses of randomized control trials and recommendations of clinical experts: treatment for myocardial infarction. *JAMA.* **268**(2): 240–8.

4   Eddy DM (1993) Three battles to watch in the 1990s. *JAMA.* **270**(4): 520–6.

CHAPTER TWO

Evidence-based practice

What do we mean by 'evidence-based clinical practice?' Evidence-based clinical practice describes the complex process of decision making and places it in the context of basing decisions on a systematic appraisal of the best evidence available (Figure 2.1). It requires a number of skills:

- the ability to define criteria such as effectiveness, safety and acceptability
- the ability to find the evidence
- the ability to assess the quality of the evidence
- the ability to assess whether the results of the research are generalisable or applicable to the whole population from which the subjects have been drawn
- the ability to assess whether the results of the research are applicable to the local situation.

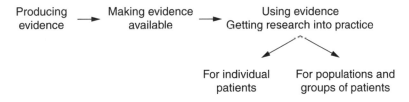

Figure 2.1: The process of evidence-based clinical practice.

The challenge for evidence-based pharmacy is twofold. The first task is to develop evidence-based medicine skills for use in clinical pharmacy whether in the secondary care setting on the ward or in primary care dealing with patients who present with problems or issues surrounding prescribed medicines.

The second part of the challenge is to find the evidence to support existing practice and to inform practice developments.

Evidence-based medicine

Much has been written on this subject, but two definitions are useful. The first is from Professor David Sackett[2]:

> Evidence-based medicine is the conscientious, explicit and judicious use of current best evidence in making decisions about the care of individual patients.

The authors go on to state that the practice of evidence-based medicine requires the integration of individual clinical expertise with the best available external clinical evidence from systematic research.

The second definition, from McKibbon,[3] is to be found on the Internet:

> Evidence-based medicine is an approach to health care that promotes the collection, interpretation and integration of valid, important and applicable patient-reported, clinician-observed and research-derived evidence. The best available evidence, moderated by patient circumstances and preferences, is applied to improve the quality of clinical judgments.

Sackett's definition deals with the criticism that evidence-based medicine is somehow a cookbook approach, as some of its critics have argued. Clinical expertise is required by clinician and pharmacist alike; the challenge is to integrate that expertise with the best evidence available. The McKibbon definition starts from the stance of collating the evidence and then applying it in the clinical setting moderated by patient circumstances and preferences. One example concerns non-steroidal anti-inflammatory drugs (NSAIDs). There is good evidence (illustrated later) to show that NSAIDs are potent analgesics in the acute pain setting, certainly better than paracetamol, dihydrocodeine or codeine, yet they are not without risk. It would be rash to use this class of drugs in a patient who is drifting into acute renal failure or who reported a history of gastric ulceration. The medicine that can provide the best outcome has to be considered in the context of the individual patient.

All this raises the question of what constitutes evidence. Table 2.1, adapted from the cancer pain guidelines developed by the US Agency for Health Care Policy and Research,[4] usefully classifies evidence into five categories.

Table 2.1 Type and strength of efficacy evidence[5]

I   Strong evidence from at least one systematic review of multiple well-designed RCTs
II Strong evidence from at least one properly designed RCT of appropriate size
III Evidence from well-designed trials without randomisation, single group pre-post, cohort, time series or matched case-controlled studies
IV Evidence from well-designed non-experimental studies from more than one centre or research group
V   Opinions of respected authorities, based on clinical evidence, descriptive studies or reports of expert committees

Evidence-based pharmacy practice

While systematic reviews about pharmacist interventions are starting to appear (*see* Chapter 9),[6] good evidence is hard to find, when classified according to Table 2.1. Pharmacists have certainly written much type V evidence but type I or II is hard to find.

Pharmaceutical care, defined by Hepler and Strand[7] as 'the responsible provision of drug therapy for the purpose of achieving definite outcomes that improve a patient's quality of life', has gained wide acceptance and is often discussed, yet the concept of pharmaceutical care has been poorly researched. There are now over 5000 articles on this subject, but the majority offer little more than opinions or accounts of activities involving small numbers of practitioners or patients. The demand for evidence to support both activity and development could cause problems for the pharmacy profession unless there is a realignment to ensure that the research currently taking place is strengthened to produce evidence that is of a higher quality. Such changes are neither difficult nor expensive in most settings, and much current research would easily lend itself to randomisation with a consequential reduction of bias.

The well-informed patient

Patients are becoming increasingly knowledgeable about their own conditions and the treatment options available for their diseases, encompassing both conventional and unconventional medicine. A great deal of information has always been available, for example through local libraries and the many patient-support groups that exist, particularly for the more serious, long-term or life-threatening illnesses. Recent years have seen an explosion of information through the Internet. Internet cafes and the high level of PC ownership mean that virtually everyone who wants to get on to the Internet can do so with relative ease, not just in the developed world, and email is now an increasingly common means of communication worldwide. The availability of searching facilities means that all types of information can be readily obtained. Add to this the fact that there are discussion groups for almost every conceivable subject, and there is no question for which an answer cannot be obtained, however bizarre that answer might be.

The Internet is generally non-judgemental; patients can ask the most trivial of questions and someone will be happy to answer. Unfortunately, the information usually comes without a quality rating, and so requires some careful interpretation. This aspect has caused some professionals to avoid the Internet, but the scenario is no different from that in the local bookshop. Any search on the shelves of a medical bookshop will reveal a wide range of information of very variable quality. Pharmacists who want to practise evidence-based pharmacy will be better placed to serve their clients by being aware of the potential of the World Wide Web.

In spite of all this, the patient is generally in the hands of a professional who often does not provide information for fear of appearing ignorant or because he or she is too busy. The scenario of the pharmacist simply handing over a bag of dispensed items is far more common than we may be prepared to admit. If we do not respond to the need to be providers of quality information, then others will do it for us. For example, the major supermarkets are more than willing to provide quality advice and materials on a number of diseases, including diabetes. The diabetes information includes material on the disease types, a summary of treatments available, which may include a brief description of each group of drugs, details on blood testing and of course dietary advice. As many of us do a good proportion of our shopping at supermarkets, some health experts are arguing that we should be able to obtain health advice and possibly treatment there as well. This has led, in part, to the UK initiative of walk-in treatment clinics in the high street.

What is available to patients?

A visit to a local library provided some interesting answers to this question. The Central Library in Oxford is probably typical of what is available to modern city dwellers in the UK. This library serves the needs of the population of the city of Oxford, some 115 000 people. Discussions with the librarians revealed that there is no set policy for either reference sources or books for loan, and that decisions to purchase books are made on an ad hoc basis. There are no on-line databases available, nor are there medical CD-ROMs or other evidence sources. A search of the shelves revealed some five metres of reference books, consisting of a haphazard collection of material. This included: a medical dictionary; a number of government reports around health issues, including immunisation and early prescribing analysis; a collection of odds and ends; patient information from several patient-support groups; and an up-to-date *British National Formulary*. The lending shelves, some 18 metres in length, contained a mixture of popular medicine and a large section on alternative medicine and disease-related popular medicine books – hardly an evidence-based resource for patients seeking information about their illness or treatment.

The limitations of evidence-based healthcare

An evidence-based approach provides some means for those providing healthcare to determine the best mix of services within limited resources. There is no guarantee, however, that benefits identified in the research setting can always be realised in practice without quality management.

Managers have the responsibility to ensure that healthcare under their supervision is supported by high-quality evidence and that it does more good than harm. They should ensure that the overall mix of services is that which provides the greatest benefit for the population being served. These services should be of sufficiently high standard to ensure that the benefits demonstrated in research studies are in fact realised.

The best healthcare is characterised by:

- no ineffective or harmful interventions
- the most effective interventions available for those groups of patients most likely to benefit
- services delivered at the highest possible quality.

Box 2.1   Best healthcare

- No ineffective or harmful interventions
- The most effective interventions available for those groups of patients most likely to benefit
- Services delivered at the highest possible quality

The health of a given population is determined by more than healthcare. The other factors are physical environment, social environment and lifestyle, and genetics.

Box 2.2   Determinants of health

- Social environment and lifestyle
- Physical environment
- Healthcare
- Genetics

Governments have been slow to incorporate such concepts into their thinking and so we continue to see departments such as transport and social services having no interaction with health, even though there is good evidence to show they are all important in maintaining and improving the health of a nation.

Implications for the patient and professional consultation

The scenario of the patient arriving at a consultation armed with a sheaf of information downloaded from the Internet is becoming increasingly common. Both the professional and the patient bring to the decision-making process a set of unspoken values which need to be considered. Professionals are often seeking to answer the questions they think their patients have, but equally often fail to ask the patients what is really bothering them. For example, a young female transplant patient may be more concerned about the growth of facial hair than to know how to take her cyclosporin at the correct time. She may in fact decide not to take the cyclosporin at all if the side effects cause embarrassment.

Box 2.3   Reasons for getting things wrong

- There may be no knowledge to know
- There may be knowledge not known to the practitioner
- There may be knowledge known but it cannot be easily applied to the clinical situation being addressed
- There may be knowledge known but it is wrong

Figure 2.2 illustrates some of the drivers at play in a pharmacist–patient consultation. The setting of the discussion is a particular challenge for the pharmacist. The clinical pharmacist on a ward often finds patients willing to discuss their medication problems. The situation may be different when the scene changes to the outpatient pharmacy, where a patient may have waited a long time to see the doctor, followed by a lengthy wait for the prescription to be dispensed. In this case, patients may not be interested in

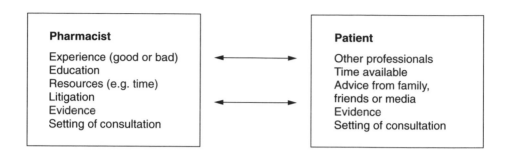

Figure 2.2: Some of the drivers at play in a pharmacist–patient interaction.

the information that needs to be conveyed. There are three elements to this communication:

1 The patient is given information.
2 The patient interprets the information.
3 The pharmacist and the patient discuss the information.

Unfortunately, the process often gets no further than step 1, and the patient then tries to remember what the important point was but has missed the valuable information that should have been understood.

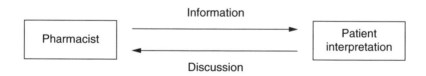

Figure 2.3: Pharmacist–patient interaction in an outpatient pharmacy.

Providing evidence-based information

The temptation in the outpatient setting and in community pharmacy is to assume a diagnosis based on the prescription. The lack of patient notes can be a real disadvantage in these situations and it may be necessary to obtain further information from the patient or the clinician involved in care. In the ward setting, the pharmacist has access to the patient's notes, which may contain information such as a serious diagnosis which the patient has not requested and does not wish to know. Obviously both these situations require careful handling. The pharmacist has a duty of care to ensure that information provided to patients is backed up by reliable sources and evidence. This applies equally to the patient who requires a 'stronger' analgesic for a minor injury or for advice for complex and potentially toxic treatment regimens. There may also be a need to reinforce information provided by other professionals involved in the patient's care.

Patients will often get their information from a number of sources, including the media. New drugs are often featured on news bulletins, and medical advice is freely offered in the newspaper supplements and magazines. New arrivals on the inpatient ward may get advice from their fellow patients on the relative merits of the analgesics, hypnotics or aperients available. In these situations, it is really important to have the evidence available. Clinical ignorance is perhaps acceptable when there is no knowledge to be known, but not so if the knowledge is available but unknown to the practitioner.

Interpretation

Once the information has been given to a patient, he or she has to interpret it and may need some time to consider it. Written material may be important, both on a label and as additional information. It is professionally unacceptable to label a medicine 'as directed', even if that is how the surgery issued the prescription, without first ensuring that the patient knows what this means and is aware of usual or maximum doses where appropriate. Medicines are often labelled in a form of words that is not readily understood by a significant proportion of the population. Some of the stock phrases require some explanation, such as 'Avoid alcohol' or 'This medicine may cause drowsiness; if affected do not drive or operate machinery'.

Discussion

The quality of the discussion will be determined by the relationship between the patient and the practitioner. An appropriate platform for this discussion to take place is often an explanation of the medicines and provision of some further relevant information.

Practising evidence-based clinical pharmacy

Building on the definition of evidence-based medicine quoted at the beginning of this chapter, it is possible to define evidence-based

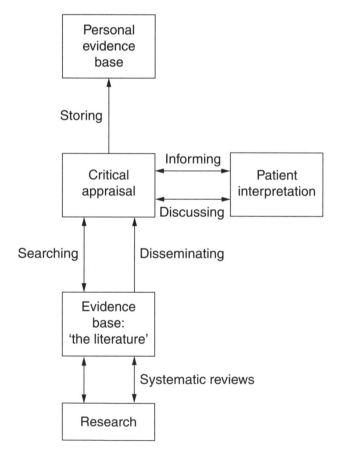

Figure 2.4: Practising evidence-based clinical pharmacy.[1]

clinical pharmacy as the conscientious, explicit and judicious use of current best evidence when making decisions about individual patients. The use of the word 'judicious' signifies that the pharmacist must take into account the patient's condition, values and circumstances.

Evidence and the pharmaceutical industry

The pharmaceutical industry in general has been slow to pick up on the evidence-based medicine movement, although attitudes are now changing and a number of companies are wanting to become involved. The approaches outlined above need to permeate the whole of the management of medicines and there is much for the industry to note.

Drug development

The industry is extremely innovative in many areas of medicines development, yet efforts are still geared to the need for registration. There are few examples where the industry has made use of measures of effectiveness such as numbers needed to treat (NNTs) or robust cost-effectiveness, and this has caused problems for the introduction of some new and expensive treatments where drugs have not been sufficiently effective to be perceived as providing value for money.

In discussing the problems of working with the results of clinical trials, in a lecture delivered some 25 years ago, Sheiner[8] listed three diseases of clinical drug evaluation. They are still relevant today.

- An irrelevant analysis. There is still a strong emphasis on the question 'Does the drug work?' rather than on 'How well does the drug work?'. This leads to emphasis on finding a dose that is effective. There are examples in recent years of drugs that have come to market with a recommended dose which has subsequently been reduced when it has been discovered that lower doses produce similar responses and fewer side effects.
- A great waste. Sheiner reports that 18 000 people were studied

in the work-up for cimetidine to gain marketing approval. The trial was designed around the need to reject the null hypothesis, even though this approach ignores the whole spectrum of patients in a real world of clinics and surgeries – the young, the old, the renally compromised, those on multiple therapy, etc. This results in narrow indications being licensed and means important groups in society who need treatment, such as children, often have to be treated outside existing product licences at the discretion of practitioners.

- Sheiner's third disease is that of an excessive conservatism caused by an emphasis on intention-to-treat analysis. He asks if it is the drug itself or the intention to treat which has efficacy. He questions the whole philosophy of this practice used in the statistics of clinical trials.

Evidence is very important at the marketing stage and the days of the glossy brochure with pretty graphs and unlabelled axes are numbered, if not past. Sadly, many clinicians and pharmacists around the world gain their knowledge from the 'drug rep'. The industry sees the rep or drug detailer as an important part of their sales strategy. In the UK, there is one pharmaceutical company representative for every six GPs. Many companies regulate the behaviour of their representatives by setting sales targets and providing incentives. It is not surprising that some reps use a variety of measures to achieve those results, and companies have little control over what happens in the field. An extreme example led to a notable quotation from a drug rep working in Bombay,[9] who stated that he worked on the principle of three 'C's for persuading clinicians to prescribe. 'My strategy is to first try to convince the doctor to support the product. If that doesn't work, I try to confuse the doctor by filling him with unnecessary technical details. If nothing else, this at least generates some curiosity in the product. If I don't succeed in this too, then I try to corrupt him. A generous quota of samples, expensive gifts, invitation to cocktail parties and what not from the company often does the job.'

Of course we may argue that the developed world has left these tactics behind and all is controlled by codes of practice. There have been some studies around these issues, and one interesting piece of work carried out as a Master's thesis in Australia[10] would suggest all is not as sound as we might like to think. There is a clear indication that while representatives provided information on indications, dosage and administration, minimal information was provided in other areas, particularly those associated with product risk. Presentations were often not judged to be balanced and were found to contain inaccuracies. The study was carried out in Melbourne and a sample of medical practitioners were asked to audio-tape their encounters with pharmaceutical representatives as well as complete a one-page questionnaire for each interview. The study had ethical approval and both the GP involved and the representative were required to complete a consent form. The representative was given time both to read the consent letter and to discuss this with the GP prior to agreeing to take part. The author recognised that it was difficult to get a representative sample from this approach and that the presence of recording could have led to an improved practice from the pharmaceutical rep. The recordings, all made one to one, were then transcribed and analysed.

Seven GPs (out of 15 invited) made some 16 recordings. Twenty four reps were asked to participate, and 16 agreed. The recordings covered 14 different pharmaceutical companies and, on average, four drugs were presented (range one to 14) in each encounter. The average length of interviews was almost 13 minutes (range four to 32 minutes). Several interesting points emerge from this small study. For example, 73% of the words are spoken by the reps. A number of inaccuracies against approved product information were recorded. In some cases, the information was clearly wrong, for example (correct answers are in brackets):

- Oestradiol patches. Rep: 'It's not metabolised by the liver' (mainly liver metabolism).
- Azelic acid. Rep: 'You can use this product and go out into the sun. There is no photosensitivity' (*BNF* side effects: rarely photosensitivity but it does exist).

Anecdotal evidence was used to support claims in six encounters. For example, one rep is quoted as saying 'I used it (oral steroid combination) for a while. It really is very good, I think'. Another regarding the appetite suppressant dexflenfluramine (no longer available): 'The patients report that they stop at the second chocolate biscuit now ... instead of the eighth or ninth'.

Many practitioners use the pharmaceutical company representative as a source of drug information, yet in this study the following problems were encountered:

- Information was only provided on indications, dosage, administration and availability.
- There was little, if any, information on contraindications, warnings, adverse drug reactions or special groups.
- Omission of risk information was most obvious.
- Thirteen of the 33 details contained at least one inaccuracy.
- Product comparisons were often used and the competitor product was displayed in a way that was not helpful.

The World Health Organisation (WHO) advocates the provision of factual and supportable information for appropriate drug use as a right for health workers and consumers. It also supports balanced information provision where positive claims must be balanced by information on side effects, contraindications and warnings.

Medico-legal implications

Iain Chalmers, Director of the UK Cochrane Centre, argues that patients should sue when available research is not put into practice.[11] He reiterates the issue that health authorities and trusts have a duty to seek the relevant information for themselves and not to expect it to come down the line as if by magic.

Evidence is a term widely used in the legal system and it is likely that the concept of evidence-based medicine will influence medico-legal claims. Interventions will need to show that they are supported by 'a reasonable body of medical opinion', and there will also be a need to show that procedures and protocols are firmly underpinned with quality evidence.

References

1   Gray JAM (1997) *Evidence-based Health Care: how to make health policy and management decisions.* Churchill Livingston, Glasgow.

2   Sackett D, Rosenberg W, Muir Gray JA, Haynes B, Scott Richardson W (1996) Evidence based medicine: what it is and isn't. *BMJ*, **312**: 71–2.

3   McKibbon KA *et al.* (1998) The medical literature as a resource for evidence based care [Web page]. Available at hiru.mcmaster.ca/hiru/medline/mdl-ebc.htm

4   Jacox A, Carr DB, Payne R *et al.* (1994) *Management of Cancer Pain*. Clinical Practice Guideline No 9. AHCPR Publication No. 94-0592. Agency for Health Care Policy and Research, US Dept of Health and Human Services, Public Health Service, Rockville, MD.

5   Moore A, McQuay H, Gray JAM (1995) Bandolier, *The First 20 issues*. NHS R&D, Oxford.

6   Bero LA, Mays NB, Barjeteh K, Bond C (1998) Expanding outpatient pharmacists' roles and health services utilisation, costs, and patient outcomes. In: *The Cochrane Library*. Update Software, Oxford.

7   Hepler CD, Strand LM (1990) Opportunity and responsibilities in pharmaceutical care. *Am J Hosp Pharm*. **47**(3): 533–43.

8   Sheiner LB (1991) The intellectual health of clinical drug evaluation. *Clin Pharmacol Ther*. **50**(1): 4–9.

9   Kamat VR, Nichter M (1997) Monitoring product movement: an ethnographic study of the pharmaceutical sales representatives in Bombay, India. In: Bennett S, McPake B, Mills A, *Private Health Providers in Developing Countries: serving the public interest?* Zed Books, London & New Jersey.

10 Roughead E (1995) The pharmaceutical representative and medical practitioner encounter: implications for quality use of medicines. MSc thesis [Web page]. Available at www.camtech.com.au/~malam/reps/tindex.htm

11 Chalmers I (1998) Patients should sue when available research isn't put into practice. *Health Service Journal*. **108**:18.

CHAPTER THREE

Asking the right questions

The journal *Bandolier*[1] asks three questions as part of its title logo:

- What do we think?
- What do we know?
- What can we prove?

All three questions are important, and the role of evidence-based practice is to move us on from the first through the second to the third, what we can prove. Much of what happens in healthcare is based on what we think. The opinions we own are derived from our mentors, our own reading or experience. For example, many pharmacists know that the treatment for night cramp is quinine. They will not have read an up-to-date paper or meta-analysis (although one exists[2]), but have acquired this knowledge at some stage in their career. Some will have an opinion on the correct dose and whether treatment should be continuous or not. In reality, the evidence is very flimsy. The meta-analysis covers only 107 patients studied across six clinical trials. While quinine was found to reduce the number of cramps compared to placebo, it did not reduce the severity or duration of cramps.

Gathering knowledge

Many pharmacists maintain a file of useful articles gathered over a period of time. These can be a good starting point, but suffer from various shortcomings. The file will certainly be incomplete, what is in the file has probably come from at least some biased sources and the information is likely to be fairly random in terms of its accumulation.

Some pharmacists will regularly acquire information by use of one or more bibliographic databases, but many wrongly believe that this facility is only available to specialist librarians. Medline is now available for Internet searching from a number of provider sites and can be accessed without charge by anyone with Internet access. *International Pharmaceutical Abstracts* is one of the most useful databases for pharmacy but is difficult to obtain. From time to time some of the popular internet providers, e.g. AOL, provide free access to this database.

The following may help those who are not familiar with using Medline or other databases.

- Medline refers to the electronic version of *Index Medicus, International Nursing Index* and *Index to Dental Literature*.
- Other names are commonly used as synonyms for Medline but refer to the search software that is used by commercial organisations licensed by the US National Library of Medicine.
- When looking for articles in the clinical literature via a computer, one of these is commonly used: Silver Platter, Ovid (formerly CD Plus) or Knowledge Finder. In all cases, the content is the same, namely the National Library of Medicine Medlars database. They are not different versions of Medline, but they may access the data in different ways.
- Ovid Technologies and Silver Platter are the two major suppliers in the UK. They have each developed their own software (Ovid for Ovid Technologies and Spirs or WinSpirs or MacSpirs for Silver Platter) for accessing Medline. If you have access to one of the dial-in facilities then it is likely that one of these packages will also be used as the access software.

Other databases

Although Medline is fairly comprehensive for clinical enquiries, it has a strong US bias and may not be the best source of references when looking for wider topics or other aspects of healthcare. There are other more appropriate databases for different areas, namely

HealthPlan for health management, and CINAHL (Cumulative Index to Nursing and Allied Literature) for nursing and the allied professions. Embase (the electronic version of the printed *Excerpta Medica*) has a better coverage of European journals and also includes more references to drugs and therapeutics articles. *International Pharmaceutical Abstracts* covers a wide range of pharmacy and pharmacology. There is a great deal of overlap between these databases, but as no single one can deliver a complete picture, several often need to be used.

What is the best way to search?

The most important stage of any search is deciding and defining exactly what needs to be found – it is important therefore to avoid just typing in the first word that comes to mind. The query needs to be formulated in terms of a question and then broken down into the component concepts. This helps to clarify the search and improve the yield of the search.

MeSH

The National Library of Medicine indexes every article included in Medline, using a controlled list of words known as a thesaurus. This list is called the Medical Subject Headings list or MeSH for short. The authors of MeSH made a deliberate choice of the terms to be used; for example, the preferred term for kidney disease is 'kidney diseases' not 'renal diseases'. For most entries, there will be broader, narrower and related terms. When searching for good-quality evidence it is important not to miss out on what could be key references, and so deciding on the best term or terms to use is critical. There is an advantage to searching with MeSH terms – because the index term describes the content of the paper, the search will pick up those papers which are about the subject under examination, even if neither title nor abstract contains the subject word.

It is also important to make sure that all the relevant indexing terms are included and that the search has not been inadvertently limited. It is possible to explode MeSH terms. When a MeSH term is 'exploded', it means that the software will search for all the papers that have been indexed with the narrower concepts that are included under the broader term. One example of the use of MeSH terms is that a search for the term 'heart disease', when exploded, includes papers on arrhythmia.

Both Ovid and Silver Platter include the MeSH terms in their search package. Ovid will automatically map the word you type into a MeSH term. You can also have a look at the MeSH preferred terms by clicking on 'tools' in the bar at the top of the screen. Silver Platter has a thesaurus option that contains the MeSH terms. In addition, the National Library of Medicine publishes books of MeSH terms showing how they explode and what is covered under each one. This is a useful resource to access from time to time for complex searches. These books of MeSH terms are available in medical libraries and the terms are also listed on the *Cochrane Library* CD-ROM.

'Boolean operators'

Although all commercial providers of Medline cater for 'natural language' queries to a greater or lesser extent, a more effective search can be carried out by using the MeSH terms that have been selected and combining these with the logical connectors OR and AND. Thus in undertaking a search around nutrition of the elderly, the terms that would need to be chosen are 'nutrition' and the related terms 'diet', 'food' and 'food habits'. By combining these terms with the connector OR, all the papers indexed under nutrition as well as all those that have been indexed under diet, food or food habits will be identified. It is then important to limit the search to only those papers which concern old people by using the connector AND and the term 'aged'. For example:

- #1 'nutrition' OR 'diet' OR 'food' OR 'food habits'
- #2 #1 AND 'aged'.

It needs to be remembered that the personnel who carry out indexing are human and they can make mistakes and omissions. To be absolutely sure of achieving as many published papers as possible, i.e. that your search has maximum sensitivity, you should search using not only MeSH terms, but also as many synonyms for your subject as you can think of that might occur in the title or abstract, for example:

- 'anemia – hypochromic' (this is a MeSH term)

OR

- 'iron deficiency anaemia' (this is a natural language phrase).

In this example, note that anaemia is spelt differently in the US and UK.

Using Medline to find the evidence

The evidence-based world seems to be one where information is often readily shared, thus making life considerably easier for everyone. A website in Oxford (www.ihs.ox.ac.uk/library/filters.htm) now has a series of search filters available for download to ensure that the hit rate is the best possible when searching for different types of evidence. There is a plan to work up further examples for use with Embase, CINAHL and PsycLit.

There are series of filters for either Silver Platter or Ovid front ends and the following are available:

- systematic review search strategies
- RCT search strategies
- diagnosis methodological filter
- prognosis methodological filter
- therapy methodological filter
- aetiology, causation or harm methodological filter
- guidelines methodological filter
- treatment outcome methodological filter
- evidence-based healthcare methods filter.

These have all been developed using appropriate expertise from the UK Cochrane Centre, NHS Centre for Reviews and Dissemination, Clearing House for Health Outcomes, School of Health and Related Research Sheffield (ScHARR) and McMaster University. Using these filters greatly improves the search yield.

Other useful sources

The *Cochrane Library* is becoming an increasingly valuable source of knowledge with over 1000 systematic reviews and approaching 300 000 RCTs. In addition, there are reviews from the Dare database (Database of Reviews of Effectiveness) produced by the NHS Centre for Reviews and Dissemination in York.

One of the important aspects, which will be illustrated later, is to ensure that a real attempt is made to find all the evidence. If we only attempt to find one or two articles to answer our questions, we may end up with the wrong answer.

Sources useful in pharmacy

The databases mentioned above all include useful material for pharmacists. To find the evidence, a search of Medline alone is no longer sufficient. Embase should be considered as essential, although sadly it is not always easy to obtain. *International Pharmaceutical Abstracts* is excellent for pharmacy references, but can be even more difficult to source. Most of these can be obtained on CD-ROM remotely via the Internet, thus reducing expensive on-line charges, especially for large searches requiring the downloading of several hundred abstracts. Sadly, Pharmline is of little use as it is not comprehensive; it contains many articles of interest to pharmacy but these are so haphazard in selection that a search of the other databases has to be done anyway.

Potential searchers should be aware that the journals indexed in bibliographic databases are liable to change from time to time, which has several implications. First, a journal may have been added to the list relatively recently and there will have been no retrospective search of the journal prior to its entry date. Second, a journal may have changed title, and it is important to check that the journal was included under its previous title. Third, journals can sometimes drop out of the searched list simply because the publishers of the database found a more worthy journal to include.

The rise of the systematic review

Reviews have been popular for a long time because, like fast food, they provide instant satiation of a need. Equally, like fast food they can be of extremely variable quality. Reviews can be misleading for the following reasons.

- They may represent only a proportion of the literature on a subject, often because the search for articles has been inadequate. This may be for a number of reasons, including poor search terms, a failure to use a wide range of databases, and restricting the search to the English language or to a short chronological time period.
- Data are abstracted in a subjective way with no assessment of the quality of the data source.
- Poor analytical techniques were used to abstract any data, or worse, no attempt was made to bring data together.

The systematic review should exhibit the following characteristics:

- A clearly defined search strategy, outlining the search terms, the breadth of the search and the databases searched.
- Follow-up of relevant cited articles in identified papers and any hand-searching of other relevant literature.
- Explicit criteria to evaluate the quality of the papers reviewed. Various scoring systems exist. However, methods that are readily reproducible across reviewers are more difficult. An example is given as Table 3.1.
- The findings are analysed using validated methods.

Box 3.1   Common faults found in systematic reviews

- Literature search incomplete
- Bias to language, usually English
- No attempt to assess quality of included studies
- Poor analytical techniques
- Conclusions not consistent with results

Table 3.1 Scoring system to evaluate the quality of papers reviewed[3]

	Score
Is the study randomised?	
Yes	1
Is the randomisation appropriate	
Yes, e.g. random number tables	1
No, e.g. alternate patients	−1
Was the study double-blind?	
Yes	1
Was blinding correctly carried out?	
Yes, e.g. double dummy	1
No, e.g. treatments did not look identical	−1
Were withdrawals and dropouts described?	
Yes	1

The table allows for a maximum score of 5.

A systematic review should seek to bring together the world literature on a subject irrespective of language of publication or date of publication. Systematic reviews of RCTs provide the highest level of evidence of efficacy of treatments, although in other circumstances, such as adverse events or diagnostic tests, randomised trials may not always provide the best evidence.

Output from systematic reviews

The evidence provided in systematic reviews can take various forms. Often it is statistical – an odds ratio, relative risk, hazard ratio or effect size. These show statistical superiority of one treatment over another, or over no treatment, but it is often difficult to relate them to clinical practice. Because of this, the concept of the NNT is increasingly being used as a useful way of looking at results of reviews or trials for at least two reasons. It is easy to calculate, and provides the treatment-specific result in a form that is understandable.

Meta-analysis

Meta-analysis is a technique used to pool the data reported in clinical trials. This method has several advantages.

- It illustrates the overall pooled effect of a number of trials that individually may show a trend that is inconclusive. The meta-analysis weights the trial size to effect, so that the pooled result gives a clear indication of whether an intervention is effective or not (*see* Figure 1.2 in Chapter 1).
- It has the effect of increasing the precision of the conclusions of a systematic review. It does this by making comparisons between several studies more objective and provides a means of dealing with results that seem to conflict.

It is important, however, that systematic reviews and meta-analyses are conducted using rigorous scientific techniques, otherwise bias can be introduced at the trial selection stage.

The meta-analysis relies on trials that have been published. The issue of unpublished trials is often raised, arguing that negative trials often remain unpublished and that if these could be included they would somehow reverse the answer delivered by the meta-analysis. A recent amnesty on unpublished data failed to produce any useful answers to this, but in many cases the amount of unpublished data would need to be enormous to counteract existing evidence that has undergone careful meta-analytic examination. Authors of good meta-analyses have normally made attempts to identify any unpublished material; however, the task is often time-consuming and largely without reward. This issue is considered further in a section on funnel plot in Chapter 4.

Why randomised trials?

The RCT is the most reliable way to assess the effect of an intervention. The principle of randomisation is simply that a subject has an equal probability of being assigned to any particular group within the study and that allocation to the group is purely chance. Randomisation eliminates selection bias by removing any influence of the investigators over assigning a subject to one group or another. It is important that the condition of being assigned to one group or another purely by chance is maintained. This could be achieved by tossing a coin, for example, but is normally delivered by either random number tables or computer-generated randomisation. Any feature that predetermines which group a subject is assigned to should be avoided. This includes the use of hospital numbers, date of birth or even the order patients were seen in the clinic list.

RCTs by their nature require that the question being asked is at a state of equipoise, i.e. of two or more treatments it is not known whether one is better than the other, and if there is a difference, which is better. It is not ethical to assign patients to treatment arms that are known to be inferior.

In addition to randomisation, bias is further eliminated by the use of blinding or masking of treatments and of the outcomes assessment. The standard approach is to double blind so that neither the investigator nor the subject knows which treatment the subject is receiving. It is important therefore that treatments are identical in appearance. Where treatments are physically different then a double-dummy technique is also required. For example, in a comparison between an injectable and an oral treatment, subjects would receive either an active injection with an oral placebo or a placebo injection with an active oral treatment. It has been shown that RCTs that do not use a double-blind design are more likely to overestimate the results. Similarly, a lack of blinding can cause the observer recording outcomes to over- or underestimate the effect of the treatment group based on pre-conceived ideas about that treatment.[4,5] The precision of the RCT increases as the number of patients in the trial increases. In fact, it is likely that studies with small samples may miss an important clinical difference that actually does exist. Equally these studies may by chance report a difference which in fact is not true.

How to develop searching skills

Everyone who is involved in decision making or is actively involved in clinical pharmacy should be able to perform the following tasks.

- Define and identify the sources of evidence to search for when faced with a particular decision.
- Carry out a search of Medline or Embase without the help of a librarian and find at least 60% of the reviews or studies that would have been found by a librarian.
- Construct simple search strategies on Medline using Boolean operators for the following:
  - healthcare terms:
    - treatment
    - screening programme
  - service elements
    - effectiveness
    - safety
    - acceptability
    - appropriateness
    - quality
    - cost-effectiveness.

There are plenty of opportunities for training, often through the nearest medical library. It is important, however, for the skills to be maintained. The skills are not only a valuable addition to any pharmacist's tool kit, but also enable published articles to be appraised more effectively.

References

1   Moore A, McQuay H, Gray JAM (1995) Bandolier, *The First 20 Issues*. NHS R&D, Oxford.

2   Man-Son-Hing M, Wells G (1995) Meta-analysis of efficacy of quinine for treatment of nocturnal leg cramps in elderly people. *BMJ*. 310: 13–17.

3   Jadad AR, Moore RA, Carroll D *et al.* (1996) Assessing the quality of reports of randomised clinical trials: is blinding necessary? *Controlled Clinical Trials*. 17: 1–12.

4   Schulz KF, Chalmers I, Hayes RJ, Altman DG (1994) Failure to conceal treatment allocation schedules in trials influences estimates of treatment effects. *Controlled Clinical Trials*. 15: 63S–64S.

5   Schulz KF, Grimes DA, Altman DG, Hayes RJ (1996) Blinding and exclusions after allocation in randomised controlled trials: survey of published paralleled group trials in obstetrics and gynaecology. *BMJ*. 312: 742–4.

CHAPTER FOUR

The tools of evidence-based medicine

One of the exciting developments around evidence-based medicine has been the emergence of new concepts that help to graphically illustrate and quantify how well a medicine works. This has brought understanding to many who failed to grasp statistics during their training and therefore have avoided any statistical analysis ever since. This chapter examines some of these new concepts.

Confidence intervals

Most pharmacists will be aware of p values in terms of an answer being significant (in a statistical sense) or not. However, use of 'p' is now largely dead and new methods of reporting significance have emerged.

As the use of the p-value has declined, so the use of the confidence interval (CI) has increased. The CI, usually set at 95% limits (although others may be used), is a visual and comprehensible way of describing the confidence that can be placed on 'the result'. By describing the CI, the range of the result can be seen clearly, in this case with a confidence of 95% that the 'result' is correct.

Confidence intervals figure largely in many systematic reviews, in meta-analyses and for describing NNTs. For example, the NNT for paracetamol in moderate or severe postoperative pain is 3.6 (3.0–4.4).[1] While it is tempting to concentrate on the single figure of 3.6, in reality the answer lies somewhere between 3.0 and 4.4.

Power

More recently there has been growing interest in the power of a study. This is described as:

> the probability that a study of a given size would detect a statistically significant real difference of a given magnitude.[2]

If the difference expected is a 100% reduction in mortality, a small study will have sufficient power. However, if the expected reduction in mortality is much smaller, say 5%, then a very much larger study must be conducted to produce a result which will have statistical significance. The question still needs to be addressed as to whether a statistical significance has any clinical relevance; it may not be of any clinical value whatsoever.

Post-hoc power

It is becoming increasingly common to ask in journal clubs or in letters to the editors of journals, 'What was the power of the study to detect the observed difference?' This may seem a sensible question to ask, but an excellent article by Goodman and Berlin[3] points out why this question is inappropriate and how to place reliance on CIs. This paper is commended to those who regularly read original trial reports.

Another important paper[4] is that by David Moher and his colleagues in Ottawa. This group reviewed 383 RCTs published in 1975, 1980, 1985 and 1990 in *JAMA*, *Lancet* and *New England Journal of Medicine*. Of these, 27% were classified as having negative results, but only a small fraction had sufficient power to detect relative differences of 25% or even 50%, and only 20 of the 102 reports made any statement related to the clinical significance of the observed differences.

Numbers needed to treat (NNTs)

The NNT is a measure of clinical significance and moves thinking from 'Does a treatment work?' to 'How well does a treatment work?' This concept is steadily gaining wide acceptance and is useful not only in its own right, but also to enable direct comparisons of treatment. The two league tables of treatments from the Oxford Pain Research Unit shown in Figures 4.1 and 4.2 illustrate the impact of such an approach. The nearer an NNT is to one, the perfect NNT, the more effective the treatment.

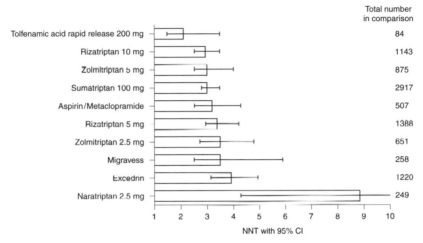

Figure 4.1: League table of NNTs for successful treatment of acute migraine attack at two hours with oral analgesics in patients with moderate to severe pain.

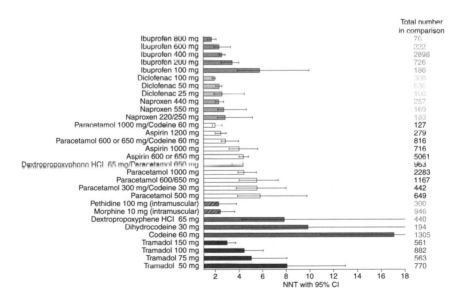

Figure 4.2: League table of NNTs to produce at least 50% pain relief over four to six hours compared to placebo in pain of moderate or severe intensity.

The NNT is usefully defined as: 'the number of people who have to be treated for one to benefit.'

Calculating the NNT

The NNT calculation is given in Figure 4.3 and is based on the understanding of risk ratios. While the NNT is the reciprocal of the absolute risk reduction, it is not necessary to understand this concept to calculate NNTs. To help, a worked example is included so that the process is transparent. The equation is quite simple; once grasped, it is easy to calculate NNTs from published trials using a pocket calculator.

	Controls	Actives
Number of patients	N_{con}	N_{act}
Improved = clinical end point	Imp_{con}	Imp_{act}

$$NNT = \frac{1}{\dfrac{Imp_{act}}{N_{act}} - \dfrac{Imp_{con}}{N_{con}}}$$

Figure 4.3: Calculating the number needed to treat (NNT).

NNTs were initially used to describe prophylactic interventions.

One example is of a study looking at influenza vaccination in the elderly. The study was conducted in the winter of 1991–92 in southern Holland. Nearly 10 000 people not known to belong to a high-risk group in 15 GP practices were asked whether they wished to take part in the study and just under 2000 accepted.[5]

People were randomly allocated to active vaccine or control, which were given in double-blind conditions in weeks 44–46 (November) before a peak of influenza incidence in Holland. The active vaccine consisted of two Beijing strains, a Singapore and a Panama strain. Participants gave blood samples before vaccination, three weeks later and five months later for serological testing for increased antibody levels. The participants and their GPs also completed forms relating to any symptoms of influenza according to defined protocols. In the vaccinated population, the rate of influenza or influenza-like illness was half that in the population given a placebo vaccination. For influenza confirmed both clinically and serologically, the relative risk was 0.42 (CI 0.23 to 0.74).

Table 4.1   Results of influenza vaccine randomised controlled trial

	Number	Total in group
Contracting flu on active	41	927
Contracting flu on control	80	911

Using the more user-friendly NNT method of calculating the results, of about two cases of influenza expected each winter in every 23 people aged over 60 years, one was prevented by influenza vaccination. Preventing one case of influenza for every 23 people treated and preventing half the cases in elderly people is a very positive result, and one which should encourage the active pursuit of the policy of influenza vaccination.

The NNT for prophylaxis is given by the expression 1/(proportion benefiting from control intervention minus the proportion benefiting from experimental intervention), and for treatment by 1/(proportion benefiting from experimental intervention minus the proportion benefiting from control intervention).

It has been previously stated that NNTs for treatment should be small, ideally one; but in reality this is unlikely. When it is remembered that few treatments are 100% effective and few controls – even placebo or no treatment – are without some effect, NNTs for effective treatments are usually in the range of 2 to 4. Exceptions might be treatments such as antibiotics; the NNT for *Helicobacter pylori* eradication with triple or dual therapy, for instance, is 1.2.[6]

NNTs for prophylaxis will be larger: few patients are affected in large populations, so the difference between treatment and control will be small, giving large NNTs. For instance, use of aspirin to prevent one death at five weeks after MI had an NNT of 40.[6]

Other ways to calculate NNTs

Using absolute risk reduction

The absolute risk reduction (ARR) is the difference between the event rate in the experimental group and the event rate in the control group. It is the denominator in the NNT calculation. Many reviews and trials provide this information, so if you have it and convert it into a proportion, then you can get the NNT by dividing 1 by the ARR:

$$\text{NNT} = 1/\text{ARR}.$$

Using odds ratios

When it is legitimate and feasible to combine data, the odds ratio is the accepted statistical test to show that the experimental intervention works significantly better than the control. If a quantitative systematic review produces odds ratios but no NNTs, it is possible to derive NNTs from a table available on the *Bandolier* website.[7]

A caveat here is that odds ratios should be interpreted with caution when events occur commonly, as in treatments, and odds ratios may overestimate the benefits of an effect when event rates are above 10%. Odds ratios are likely to be superseded by relative risk reduction (RRR) because RRR provides better information in situations where event rates are high.[8]

Relative risk reduction

Chatelier and colleagues[9] have published a useful NNT nomogram (Figure 4.4). RRR – the percentage reduction in risk between the experimental and control groups – is used to calculate the NNT for any group in which the risk of an event happening was known. This is probably most likely to be used in prophylaxis. Provided that a review or paper gives a RRR (in per cent) and that it is possible to determine the susceptibility of a patient to a bad outcome (usually called the 'patient expected event rate' or PEER), then it is possible to find out the NNT of an intervention. RRR is calculated by dividing the difference between the rate of events in the experimental and control groups by the rate of events in the control group. So if 10% of patients have a bad event in controls, and only 9% with some intervention, the RRR is $(10 - 9)/10 = 10\%$. RRRs happen in prophylaxis. With treatments, relative risk increases are reported because there will be more good events. The method works either way.

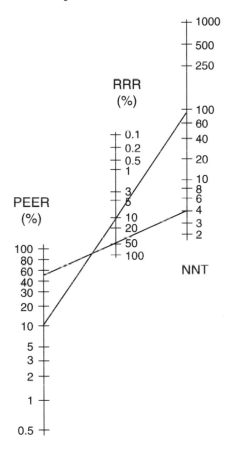

Figure 4.4: Nomogram for NNTs.

If the RRR in Figure 4.4 is 50%, and the PEER is 50%, then the NNT from the nomogram is 4. But if the RRR is 10% and the PEER is 10%, then the NNT is about 90.

How can NNTs help decision making?

First, NNTs help make decisions between treatment options, and this is where most systematic reviews are useful. If the NNT for treatment A is lower (better) than that for treatment B, then, all other things being equal, choosing A over B makes sense. There are, of course, many nuances to all this. These are outlined in a book from David Sackett and colleagues entitled *Evidence-based Medicine: how to practise and teach evidence-based medicine.*[10] This book is a valuable addition to any practice bookshelf.

L'Abbé plots

A paper[11] by Kristen L'Abbé and colleagues written in 1987 is an extremely valuable contribution to understanding systematic reviews and is perhaps one of the most sensible and understandable papers on this topic. The authors suggest a simple graphical representation of the information from trials. Each point on a L'Abbé scatter plot represents one trial in the review. The proportion of patients achieving the outcome with the experimental intervention is plotted against the event rate in controls (Figure 4.5). Even if a review does not show the data in this way, it is relatively simple to determine this, if the information is in the review.

For treatment, trials in which the experimental intervention was better than the control will be in the upper left of the plot, between the y axis and the line of equality. If experimental was no better than control then the point will fall on the line of equality, and if control was better than experimental then the point will be in the lower right of the plot, between the x axis and the line of equality.

For prophylaxis this pattern will be reversed. Because prophylaxis reduces the number of bad events – such as the use of aspirin reducing death after MI – we expect a smaller proportion harmed with treatment than with control. So if experimental is better than control, the trial results cloud should be between the x axis and the line of equality.

These plots give a quick indication of the level of agreement among trials. If the points are in a consistent cloud, that gives some confidence that there is a homogenous effect. But if points

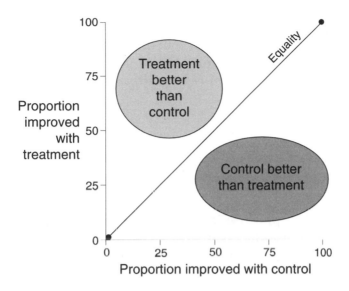

Figure 4.5: L'Abbé plot for treatment.

are spread all over the graph, and especially if they cross the line of equality, it should raise concern about the intervention, or the patients being treated and their condition. This can also be called heterogeneity.

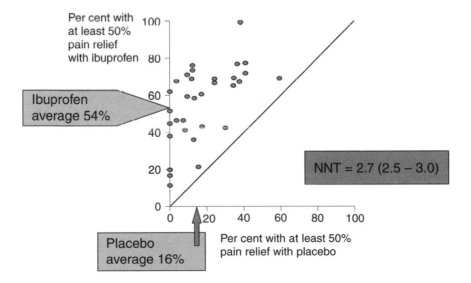

Figure 4.6: L'Abbé plot for treatment with 400 mg ibuprofen.

The important point about a L'Abbé plot is that it shows all of the extant data on one piece of paper. When combined with numbers in the trial, and a summary measure like NNT, it is a useful way to summarise a lot of information (Figure 4.6).

Using NNTs

Variation in treatment and control

One of the things that plotting information from systematic reviews in L'Abbé plots demonstrates is just how variable the effects of both treatment and control in randomised trials are. It is legitimate to be surprised, but after quite a short time it seems that this is the norm. The reasons are probably complex, but much of the variability will be just random chance. In many circumstances, patients can have quite wide patterns of response to a treatment, but trial size for treatments is often relatively small because trials can be difficult to conduct and gaining large numbers of patients in some areas of medicine is very difficult. Gathering data in systematic reviews and meta-analysis gives much more power than a single trial in almost all circumstances, especially for reviews of treatments. Seeing such variability also teaches caution when faced with a single trial with apparently excellent (or hopeless) results.

There will be circumstances where systematic reviews will not yield information to generate L'Abbé plots, NNTs, relative risks or even odds ratios. There are times when the information for quantitative systematic review is just not available; but when it is, the information is extremely useful in practising clinical pharmacy.

Can NNTs be used to inform patients?

This is a difficult area because a NNT is treatment-specific; it will not include all the power of an intervention – a placebo response, for instance. Patients want to know their chance of getting better or being harmed, and that includes influences from all sources. The best analgesics have NNTs of 2 for at least 50% pain relief (a high hurdle), which implies that half the patients will achieve at least 50% pain relief because of the analgesic. But the placebo effect will add perhaps another 20% to this, so the reality is that 70% achieve at least 50% pain relief with the analgesic, which sounds better and reflects the reality. This is a simple example, and most circumstances are more complex. The LBHH (likelihood of being helped or harmed) has been suggested as one way of presenting information to patients,[12] but there is a clear need for more empirical research to provide evidence on how best to do this.

What is an odds ratio?

The NNT is a very useful way of describing the benefits (or harms) of treatments, both in individual trials and in systematic reviews. Although few papers report results using this easily interpretable measure, NNT calculations come second to working out whether an effect of treatment in one group of patients is different from that found in the control groups. Many studies, and particularly systematic reviews, report their results as odds ratios, or as a reduction in odds ratios, and some trials do the same. Odds ratios are also commonly used in epidemiological studies to describe the likely harm an exposure might cause.

Jon Deeks[13] from the Oxford Centre for Statistics in Medicine has some useful hints.

Calculating the odds

The odds of an event are calculated as the number of events divided by the number of non-events. For example, on average, 51 babies in every 100 births are boys, so the odds of any randomly chosen delivery being that of a boy is: number of boys (51) / number of girls (49), or about 1.04. We could also have calculated this as the ratio of the baby being a boy (0.51) to it not being a boy (0.49).

If the odds of an event are greater than one, the event is more likely to happen than not (the odds of an event that is certain to happen are infinite). If the odds are less than one, the chances are that the event won't happen (the odds of an impossible event are zero).

An odds ratio is calculated by dividing the odds in the treated or exposed group by the odds in the control group. Epidemiological studies generally try to identify factors that cause harm – those with odds ratios greater than one.

For example, if we look at case-control studies investigating the potential harm of giving high doses of calcium channel blockers for hypertension, clinical trials typically look for treatments which reduce event rates, and which have odds ratios of less than one. In these cases, a percentage reduction in the odds ratios is often quoted instead of the odds ratio. For example, the ISIS-4 trial reported a 7% reduction in the odds of mortality with captopril, rather than reporting an odds ratio of 0.93.

Relative risks

Few people have a natural ability to interpret event rates that are reported in terms of odds ratios. Understanding risks and relative risks seems to be something easier to grasp.

The risk (or probability) of having a boy is simply 51/100, or 0.51. If, for some reason, we were told that the risk had doubled (relative risk = 2) or halved (relative risk = 0.5), our perception of what this would mean is that the event would be twice as likely or half as likely to occur.

Risks and odds

In many situations in medicine, we can get a long way in interpreting odds ratios by pretending that they are relative risks. When events are rare, risks and odds are very similar. For example, in the ISIS-4 study 2231 of 29022 patients in the control group died within 35 days: a risk of 0.077 [2231/29022] or an odds of 0.083 [2231/(29022 − 2231)]. This is an absolute difference of 6 in 1000 or a relative error of about 7%. This close approximation holds when we talk about odds ratios and relative risks, providing the events are rare.

Why use an odds ratio rather than relative risk?

If odds ratios are difficult to interpret, why don't we always use relative risks instead? Many academics agree and have argued that there is no place for describing treatment effects in clinical trials using odds ratios. However, they continue to be used, especially in systematic reviews.

There are several reasons for this, most of which relate to the superior mathematical properties of odds ratios. Odds ratios can always take values between zero and infinity, which is not the case for relative risk. Some readers may have already spotted a problem in the sex ratio example cited above: if the baseline risk of having a boy is 0.51, it is not possible to double it!

The range that relative risk can take therefore depends on the baseline event rate. This could obviously cause problems if we were performing a meta-analysis of relative risks in trials with greatly different event rates. Odds ratios also possess a symmetrical property: if you reverse the outcomes in the analysis and look at good outcomes rather than bad, the relationships will have reciprocal odds ratios. This again is not true for relative risks.

Odds ratios are always used in case-control studies where disease prevalence is not known: the apparent prevalence there depends solely on the ratio of sampling cases to controls, which is totally artificial. To use an effect measure which is altered by prevalence in these circumstances would obviously be wrong, so odds ratios are the ideal choice. This provides the historical link with their use in meta-analyses: the statistical methods that are routinely used are based on methods first published in the 1950s for the analysis of stratified case-control studies. Meta-analytical methods are now available which combine relative risks and ARRs, but more caution is required in their application, especially when there are large variations in baseline event rates.

A fourth point of convenience occurs if it is necessary to make adjustments for confounding factors using multiple regression. When measuring event rates the correct approach is to use logistic regression models which work in terms of odds, and report effects as odds ratios. This means odds ratios are likely to be in use for some time, so it is important to understand how to use them. Of course, it is also important to consider the statistical significance of an effect as well as its size. As with relative risks, it is easy to spot statistically significant odds ratios by noting whether their 95% CIs do not include 1, which is analogous to there being less than a 1 in 20 chance (or a probability of less than 0.05, or gambling odds of better than 19 to 1) that the reported effect is solely due to chance.

The funnel plot

The funnel plot has arisen as a technique for detecting bias in meta-analyses. We have argued that systematic reviews or meta-analyses are the best strategy for appraising and reporting evidence. There have been situations, however, where a meta-analysis has been contradicted by a later large randomised trial. It has been argued that this has arisen because of publication bias and other biases used in the process of finding, selecting and combining studies.

For example, many reviews, and this is particularly true of pharmacy reviews, have concentrated almost entirely on English-language publications. It is argued that negative findings are more likely to be published in smaller, often non-English-language, journals (even though the result is important) or in some cases do not get published at all. A useful publication by Egger and Davey Smith[14] describes a number of examples and is a good reference on the subject of bias and funnel plots. Furthermore, positive studies may be published more than once and have the potential to skew results for the unwary reviewer. A funnel plot aims to plot the trial's effect estimate against sample size and relies on the hypothesis that precision in the underlying treatment effect will increase as the sample size of the individual studies increases. Results from small studies will be scattered widely at the bottom of the graph and the spread narrows as the study size increases. If there is no bias, the graph resembles an inverted funnel (hence the name), and if it is skewed and asymmetrical this is seen as an indication of bias. An example is shown as Figure 4.7. Each dot represents a single clinical trial of a topical NSAID versus placebo.

There is an argument particularly used by opponents of systematic reviews, that a large number of unpublished trials could refute a systematic review's findings. Villar *et al.* analysed 38 meta-

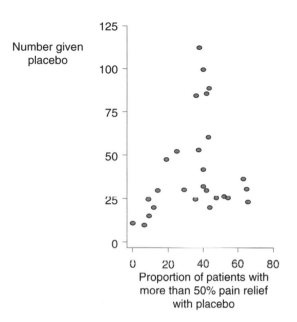

Figure 4.7:   Relationship between placebo response and trial size for topical NSAID studies of acute pain.

analyses which were reported in the pregnancy and childbirth module of the *Cochrane Library*.[15] The authors concluded that in 80% of the meta-analyses, the results were in agreement with results from large trials. In practice, it is extremely unlikely that these unpublished trials do in fact exist, and if they did they probably would not seriously change our current results.

It was stated above that the funnel plot concept is based on the hypothesis that if there is no bias then the plot is symmetrical. This aspect is currently being challenged, particularly by mathematical modelling methods. It may be that other factors are at play and the hoped-for symmetrical plots may not be so easy to obtain.

QALYs, quality-adjusted life years

Many have been perplexed at the concept of quality-adjusted life year (QALY), a slightly strange concept increasingly turning up in the literature. Ceri Phillips' 'simple' guide to QALYs[16] is as follows.

Outcomes

Outcomes from treatments and other health-influencing activities have two basic components – the quantity and quality of life. Life expectancy is a traditional measure with few problems of comparison – people are either alive or not.

However, the attempt to measure and value quality of life is a more recent innovation, with a number of approaches being used. Particular effort has gone into researching ways in which an overall health index might be constructed to locate a specific health state on a continuum between, for example, 0 (= death) and 1 (= perfect health). Obviously the portrayal of health like this is far from ideal, since the definition of perfect health, for example, is highly subjective and it has been argued that some health states are worse than death.

Uses

Construction of such measures has a number of uses – to identify public health trends so that strategies can be developed, to assess the effectiveness and efficiency of healthcare interventions or to determine the state of health in communities.

QALY calculation

The QALY has been created to combine the quantity and quality of life. The basic idea of a QALY is straightforward. It takes one year of perfect health life expectancy to be worth 1, but regards one year of less-than-perfect life expectancy as less than 1. Thus an intervention which results in a patient living for an additional four years rather than dying within one year, but where quality of life fell from 1 to 0.6 on the continuum, will generate:

- step 1: four years of extra life at 0.6 quality of life values, 2.4
- step 2: less one year at reduced quality (1 − 0.6), 0.4
- answer: QALYs generated by the intervention, 2.0.

QALYs can therefore provide an indication of the benefits gained from a variety of medical procedures in terms of quality and life and survival for the patient.

Value of QALYs

It is no use pretending that QALYs are anything but a crude measurement. It is necessary to be aware of their limitations – with the possibility that more research may make the process more sophisticated and useful. The use of QALYs in resource allocation decisions does mean that choices between patient groups competing for medical care are made explicit. QALYs have been criticised because there is an implication that some patients will be refused or not offered treatment for the sake of other patients, yet such choices have been made and are being made all the time. However big the pot, choices still have to be made.

Putting risks into perspective

Pharmacists should be able to make sense of risk or chance. There is an interesting paper[17] which suggests using the Paling perspective scale as a way of doing this.

The idea is that a scale of risk of events of interest is presented together with some ideas about risks of life events, such as being killed by lightning or in a road accident (which most of us think of as being remote), as well as more common risks. The risks of any particular event associated with a treatment can then be placed alongside, if, that is, the outcomes and timescales are generally similar. And this is something useful for irreversible events rather than adverse effects of treatment which go away when you stop taking the tablets. The graphical illustration shown in Figure 4.8 seems to be particularly valuable at getting the information across.

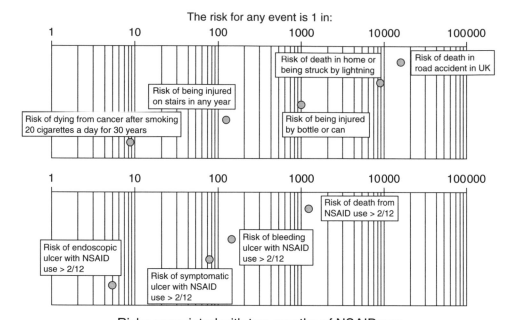

Risks associated with two months of NSAID use

Figure 4.8: Logarithmic scale of risks. Source: *Bandolier*.

References

1   Moore RA, Collins S, Carroll D, McQuay HJ (1997) Paracetamol with and without codeine in acute pain: a quantitative systematic review. *Pain.* **70:** 193–201.

2   Altman DG, Martin Bland J (1995) Absence of evidence is not evidence of absence. *BMJ.* **311:** 485.

3   Goodman SN, Berlin J *et al.* (1994) Manuscript quality before and after peer review and editing at Annals of Internal Medicine. *Ann Intern Med.* **121**(1): 11–21.

4   Moher D, Dulberg CS, Wells GA (1994) Statistical power, sample size and their reporting in randomised controlled trials. *JAMA.* **272:** 121–3.

5   Govaert Th ME, Thijs C, Masurel N, Sprenger M, Dinant G, Knottnerus J (1994) The efficacy of influenza vaccination in elderly individuals. *JAMA.* **272**(21): 1661–5.

6   Moore A, McQuay H, Gray JAM (1995) Bandolier, *The First 20 Issues*. NHS R&D, Oxford.

7   Moore RA, McQuay HJ (1997) Using odds ratios [Web page]. Available at www.jr2.ox.ac.uk/bandolier/band36/b36-2.html

8   Sinclair JC, Bracken MB (1994) Clinically useful measures of effect in binary analyses of randomised trials. *J Clin Epidemiol*. **47**: 881–9.

9   Chatelier G *et al.* (1996) The number needed to treat: a clinically useful nomogram in its proper context. *BMJ*. **312**: 426–9.

10 Sackett DL, Richardson WS, Rosenberg W, Haynes RB (1997) *Evidence-based Medicine: how to practise and teach evidence-based medicine*. Churchill Livingstone, London.

11 L'Abbé KA (1987) Meta-analysis in clinical research. *Ann Intern Med*. **107**: 224–33.

12 Chalmers I (1995) Applying overviews in meta-analysis at the bedside. *J Clin Epidemiol*. **48**: 67–70.

13 Deeks J (1996) Swots corner: what is an odds ratio? *Bandolier*. **25**: 6.

14 Egger M, Davey Smith G (1998) Meta-analysis bias in location and selection of studies. *BMJ*. **316**: 61–6.

15 Villar J, Carroli G, Belizan JM (1995) Predictive ability of meta-analyses of randomised controlled trials. *Lancet*. **345**: 772–6.

16 Phillips C (1996) So what is a QALY? *Bandolier*. **24**: 7.

17 Singh AD, Paling J (1997) Informed consent: putting risks into perspective. *Survey of Ophthalmology*. **42**: 83–6.

CHAPTER FIVE

Accessing the information

Problems with accessing the information

There is no shortage of evidence; it is estimated that there are over 30 000 medically related journals published annually.[1] If it is assumed that, on average, they all publish 100 pages per year, and some produce many more than that, then more than 3 million pages are produced annually.

The main difficulty is one of time, both to access the information and then to master it accurately. It is not easy for many practitioners to get to a good medical library, although drug information services can be very useful for tracking down material. Efficient use of readily available computer technology can be effective and time saving.

Access to information

Drug information services

Most hospital drug information services are willing to answer queries and many health authorities have a contract with a local drug information department to deal with questions from GPs, pharmacists, patients and others.

National pharmacy organisations such as the Royal Pharmaceutical Society and the National Pharmaceutical Association in the UK often have good query-answering facilities. The pharmaceutical industry is willing to answer questions about its own products and can be a useful source of papers on a particular product; the ABPI recently created an Electronic Medicines compendium which contains the information also published in the Data Sheet Compendium (summary of product characteristics).[2] Most of these agencies are set up to answer relatively simple queries in short time frames, and the question may need to be carefully composed. For example, if you are looking for quality evidence then the request needs to be for RCT or systematic review evidence. If it exists, then you should get it, but don't expect a systematic review to be undertaken for you.

Establishing access to the Internet

The Web is a great source of information and can deliver a wide range of useful material. It was estimated that in mid-1998, the Web was made up of some 320 million pages of information. In addition to having a huge range of useful services, such as travel schedules, city maps, and statistics on a wide range of topics, it also contains a vast array of useful pharmaceutical and medical material. Up-to-date treatment protocols and guidelines for a wide variety of disease states are available from many teaching hospitals in the US, for example, and a great deal of good-quality teaching material can be found for many topics. Most web browsers (software that enables exploration of the World Wide Web) are easy to use and can be accessed without charge for use. There are plenty of books to explain the Web and get you started if you prefer that method.

It may be helpful to join relevant on-line discussion groups that are able to supply useful material. If they don't work for you, discontinue membership (these are usually free and can be joined or cancelled very easily).

Build up your own list (called bookmarks or favourites) of useful Websites and visit them from time to time to see what has been updated. There is now software that can tell you when a site you are interested in has changed.

There are a number of bibliographic databases that can be searched via the Web and many of these are free, apart from any phone charges, usually at local call rates. Unfortunately this does not extend to those that have good pharmacy content, such as *International Pharmaceutical Abstracts* or Embase.

The *Cochrane Library*, which probably has the best source of RCTs, is now available on the Web for a subscription.

Attitudes to the Internet

One in two Internet users in the US spent some time looking for health information on the Internet in 1997.[3] In spite of this, professionals have generally been slow to use the Web to advantage, often hiding behind a comment that the Web is full of junk. The American Medical Association has set up a project called Physicians Accessing the Internet (PAI),[4] which has ten objectives for the physician to achieve.

- Select appropriate equipment to go on-line.
- Understand the Internet and how it works.
- Establish an Internet connection.
- Identify biomedical sources available on the Internet.
- Identify non-biomedical sources of interest available on the Internet.
- Understand basic principles of information security and communications ethics on the Internet.
- Search for needed medical information.
- Send and receive email.
- Download files, save and print as needed.
- Understand future applications of the Internet.

These are useful objectives for pharmacists wishing to become familiar with the Web.

Using the World Wide Web to best advantage

Search engines

A search engine is a sophisticated database held on a computer connected to the Web. It is accessed via one of the commonly available browsers that support the use of forms, e.g. Internet

Explorer, Netscape or Mosaic. The search engines are free, at least for the basic searches, so there is plenty of advertising to cover the costs.

The number of search engines is multiplying rapidly, so it is only possible to cover some of the more significant ones here and attempt to classify the different types. There are search engines that specialise in search engines! For example, www.thebighub. com enables over 1500 other search engines to be checked. www.metaplus.com has a more manageable selection of the better-known engines and is a useful place to start. Another site that lists hundreds of search engines in a classified way is www.search enginewatch.com; this at least enables the user to filter out those engines which are unlikely to help in providing information on medical issues.

Experts currently talk about four types of search engine:

- free text
- index-based
- meta-search
- resource- or site-specific.

Free text search engines are the easiest to use but can be hit or miss, especially if the word or phrase is somewhat ambiguous, such as the word 'trial'. Two useful examples are Alta Vista (www.altavista.com) and Northern Light (www.northern light.com), which are among my most frequently used engines.

Index-based search engines attempt to classify under certain headings, such as travel or leisure, although they may be a hybrid that seeks to provide both a free-text facility and an index. Check out www.yahoo.com, which provides around 14 major categories with three or four subcategories in each.

Meta-search engines merely enable other search engines to be searched with your query. This can save time, but the results are not quite the same as using each one in turn. This method is useful when either searching for information on a very small topic or trying to understand the scope of a topic. The two mentioned above, BigHub and Metaplus, are good examples.

Site-specific search engines enable information to be found on large Websites. A good example is the search facility on the *Bandolier* site (www.jr2.ox.ac.uk/Bandolier), which quickly finds words or terms hidden in the text of articles on the site.

Below is a list of some of the more significant search engines.

- Yahoo. One of the original search engines, it has lots of material already classified (www.yahoo.com).
- Alta Vista. Similar to Yahoo but seems to have less junk material. Claims to have indexed over 100 million Web pages, so it is probably the largest available (www.altavista. com).
- Euroseek. The site positions itself as a European portal to the Internet and enables searching to be carried out in 39 European languages (www.euroseek.com).
- Infoseek. Another of the original search engines. It has a powerful selection of search tools (www.infoseek.com).
- Lycos. This site has started offering Website reviews and has an index organised by category (www.lycos.com).
- Excite! Not as large as some of those above, but can be useful (www.excite.com).
- LookSmart (www.looksmart.com).
- HotBot (www.hotbot.com).
- Northern Light. This search engine seeks to carry out some classification of the results, so it is possible to check through a subsection that might be more relevant to the search question (www.northernlight.com).
- Global Online Directory. This one concentrates on European sites but does not seem to cover technical or educational material (www.god.co.uk).
- Ask Jeeves. Another search engine that gives a good range of response, in this case classified into basic information, specialist knowledge, purchasing sources, etc. (www.askjeeves.com).
- Mining Co. Nothing to do with mining, except that it is a mine of information. Aims to give an overview of a topic, but the quality of the commentary is variable. Recently changed to About.com (www.miningco.com).
- Starting Point. This is an index-based search engine and enables a search for a keyword or phrase on a number of other search engines. Has a health section (www.stpt.com).
- What's New Too! Again, not really a search engine, but an excellent resource for finding new sites (newtoo.manifest.com).
- WebTop. This site is useful, as it enables searches from particular types of sites or countries by using the Web address as a

filter. For example, it is possible to search looking only for those sites that include 'uk' in the Web address (www.webtop.com).
- Finally, it is worth mentioning Dogpile, a multi-engine search tool that will trawl a number of the engines mentioned above (www.dogpile.com).

Some tips for using these search tools

The size of the Web is such that no search engine can possibly hope to index all the material, but use of the engines and careful selection of links on useful sites will help. The following tips will help search out useful material.

- Seek to make the search unique by avoiding very broad search terms. Even terms like 'epilepsy' can deliver over 100 000 possible pages.
- Use the Boolean terms mentioned for searching other databases, such as 'and' or 'not'. Alta Vista allows use of the term 'near' to find related information in a section. Many search engines allow the use of single quotations for a string of words or terms such as 'pharmaceutical care'.
- Try using several engines; they do not all contain the same information and they do not all look for the information in the same way.
- If there is a news group in the subject you are looking for, check the frequently asked questions (FAQ) section.
- Choose your time carefully. The search engines are run on powerful machines but can get very busy. For example, if you are based in the UK, search the US sites in the early morning when most of the US is still asleep. The end of the day will find the computers in Australia and the Far East easier to access.

To illustrate the types of results that can be obtained, a search for the term 'diabetes' was carried out using each of the search engines noted above. The search was undertaken in July 2000 and the results are presented in Table 5.1. An arbitrary assessment of value to both patients and professionals has been made, based on a scale of one to five, five being the best.

The lessons learned from this exercise are that there is a lot of useful information but that it is not systematically organised and it

Table 5.1 Use of search engines for information on diabetes

Search engine	Search result	Value to professionals (maximum 5)	Value to patient (maximum 5)	Comment
Alta Vista	537 130 pages	2	2	Mixed bag of material. Does provide some subgroups of the subject
Ask Jeeves	8000+	2	4	Information on support groups and links to basic (encyclopaedia) type information
Dogpile	12 search engines checked. Many hits	2	3	Clinical guidelines and contacts. Mixed bag
Excite!	Number not specified but > 3000	4	4	Gives a suggested 10 'try first' sites. Listed the main ones. Excite! used by AOL (America Online) Internet provider, so often used by patients
Global Online	60 matches	0	0	Nothing of value listed
HotBot	202 500 pages	3	2	Mixed bag of hits. Lots of sites offering services to diabetics in the US
Infoseek	123 813 pages	3	1	Lots of news items and recent developments. Has additional ability to search on the pages found
LookSmart	96 matches	1	2	Some useful links to pharmaceutical industry sites with diabetes information

Table 5.1 Use of search engines for information on diabetes – *Continued*

Search engine	Search result	Value to professionals (maximum 5)	Value to patient (maximum 5)	Comment
Lycos UK	18 394 pages	2	2	Haphazard collection of pages.
Lycos Worldwide	121 097 pages			Main useful sites not in first 20 pages listed
Mining Co. (aka About.com)	1636 pages	1	1	Mixed bag of material difficult to assess
Northern Light	714 357 items	4	4	Classified into a number of useful subgroups. Searches evidence-based resources
Starting Point	54 pages	1	2	Lots of foreign-language pages
WebTop	144 784 pages	3	3	Mixed quality of hits but some useful material not seen elsewhere. Some non-English material
What's New Too!	429 hits	1	1	Little material of value
Yahoo	20 categories and 454 Websites	3	3	Lots of good-quality material sorted into groups to speed search

can be difficult to find what you need. Some rating instruments do, in fact, exist and these were reviewed by Jadad and Gagliardi.[5] The authors used a variety of methods to identify relevant information. These included a search of Medline, Cinahl and Health, a search on rating best health using six of the search engines mentioned above, and a hand search of the Internet journal world. The authors discovered 47 different rating instruments, but only 14 published the details of the rating criteria. Of these, eight appeared to be related to health information and most of these used some sort of analogue scale (stars, medals, etc.), but little information on whether the score was reached by consensus or a single observation.

In conclusion, the authors argue that the information revolution currently underway requires both scholarly discussion and rigorous evaluation and could help make healthcare more efficient and equitable, rather than it being ruled by confusion and conflict of opinions.

Specialist medical search engines

At the time of writing, several specialist medical search engines and gateways are beginning to appear. It is likely that these will provide a useful shortcut to the quality medical sites.

Scout Report Signpost (scout.cs.wisc.edu/archives/signpost.html) is a general refined resource funded by the US National Science Foundation, based at the University of Wisconsin-Madison Computer Science Department. This resource covers many areas of science, and also has a section on medicine. The site claims to contain only the best Internet resources as chosen by the editorial staff of the *Scout Report*. The site has been organised for efficient browsing but is still being developed. The hard work seems to be carried out by existing Web crawlers, and the search conducted here was routed via Excite!

Medical World Search (www.mwsearch.com) claims to be one of the first search engines on the Web especially developed for the medical field. Its aims are to provide a search engine that searches a selection of high-quality medical sites, and to allow extensive use of medical terminology via a medical thesaurus. The site is aimed at clinicians, claiming it will help them maintain their skills and inform them about new developments. It also claims to reduce the noise (useless sites and information) by using a word-statistical approach and then to selectively index medical documents from sites that are of high quality and have high clinical content. It is possible to select which Web crawler should be used and there is also an option for a Medline search. The easiest method is to select the default to 'ALL' for a wide search.

OMNI, Organising Medical Networked Information (www.omni. ac.uk), is described as a gateway to Internet resources in medicine, biomedicine, allied health, health management and related topics. It aims to provide comprehensive cover of the UK sources and link to the best international sources. OMNI is run as a consortium based at Nottingham University and funded by the Joint Information tion Systems Committee. It forms a part of the Electronic Libraries programmc (cLib).

Table 5.2 Use of medical search engines for information on diabetes

Search engine	Search result	Value to professionals (maximum 5)	Value to patient (maximum 5)	Comment
Scout Report Signpost	4	0	1	Too little material to be of value
Medsearch	3469	2	2	Material generally high-quality but some of the links and a lot of material were out of date
OMNI	74	4	4	High-quality sites including some useful guidelines

Other medical search engines include Medical Matrix, Cliniweb and MedWeb. This field is developing so rapidly that it is impossible to give a comprehensive, up-to-date listing.

Medical journal Websites

There are a good number of medical journals that offer excellent Websites. The *BMJ*, for example, has the full text of the latest edition on its Website on the morning of publication. Other journals publish either the index pages or an index with a range of complete articles, while some others provide a brief summary of their articles. This facility can be extremely valuable for journals such as *JAMA* or others not published in the UK. Some journals will deliver details of the index page to you by email for instant browsing.

Specialist pharmacy Websites

There are several pharmacy Websites. The Pharmweb site (www.pharmweb.net), based in Manchester, is quite well-known but contains little in the way of evidence. It functions largely as a signpost to other Websites. There are a few UK hospital pharmacy department Websites being set up in the UK, but the majority of good material is to be found in the US. A number of hospital sites have excellent supporting data for guidelines and protocols as well as pointers to drug information. For suggested pharmacy Websites *see* Appendix 5.

Government and NHS Websites

The Department of Health (DoH), Medicines Control Agency (MCA) and European Medicines Evaluation Agency (EMEA) all have Websites. The first can be very useful for keeping up to date with changes and legislation; for example, Government White Papers are available on the day of issue (although the Website is extremely busy when this happens!). The MCA site is somewhat devoid of useful data, but the EMEA site contains extremely useful material on new drugs that have been licensed. There is often detailed information on new drugs and discussions on the licensing that cannot easily be found elsewhere.

The NHS commissions and publishes reviews from a number of centres and some of these are now on the Web. These include DEC reports from the Development and Evaluation Committee of the former Wessex region. A number of useful evaluations can be found on the South and West Regional R&D programme of the NHS Website. The NHS Centre for Reviews and Dissemination based at the University of York publishes *Effectiveness Matters* on the Web (www.york.ac.uk/inst/crd). The National Institute for Clinical Excellence (NICE) publishes details of its workplan and also details of guidance with the underpinning evidence (www. nice.org).

Other information can be found on the NHS R&D Website (www.doh.gov.uk/research/index.htm). One of the useful features of this site is a searchable database of grants available for research.

The US government has responded to the explosion of interest in looking for health-related information on the Internet and has created a site called Healthfinder. While this site is being developed, there are the beginnings of what could be a useful first stop for consumers of healthcare (www.healthfinder.gov). The site aims to be a gateway for consumers, pointing to on-line publications, databases and support groups as well as government agencies and not-for-profit groups. The site was established in April 1997 and in the first year recorded over 1.7 million visits.

Evidence-based medicine Websites

Two useful sites that have pointers to evidence-based Websites are ScHARR, which is an excellent source of evidence sites (www.shef.ac.uk/uni/academic/R-Z/scharr/ir/netting.html), and the *Bandolier* links from the *Bandolier* pages. This site (www.jr2.ox.ac.uk/Bandolier) publishes the full text of *Bandolier*, a journal of evidence-based topics. *Bandolier* is a monthly broadsheet of evidence that is topical and a good source of NNT information. This site also contains some of the best evidence on pain relief and currently is developing evidence for a number of specialist areas including complementary medicines.

Guidelines and guidance

Several useful guideline sites exist and these include:

- Guideline (www.ihs.ox.ac.uk/guidelines/), a UK initiative to develop a database of appraised guidelines aimed at professionals within the NHS. This resource has been established by a group of four health authorities (Berkshire, Buckinghamshire, Northamptonshire and Oxfordshire) based in the NHS Executive South East Region.
- SIGN (Scottish Intercollegiate Guidelines Network). This group (www.show.scot.nhs.uk/sign/devprog.htm) has been working for some years to promote and develop good clinical practice through guideline development. Many of the guidelines are available as PDF files, which can be read using Adobe Acrobat.

A working version of the software enabling PDF files to be read is freely available via the Internet.

- AHCPR (Agency for Health Care Policy and Research). The US government publishes useful material in the form of guidelines and details of research in progress (www.nlm.nih.gov) and AHCPR is the main US agency producing national guidelines. To date some 20 guidelines have been produced and these are updated fairly regularly.

Information on CD-ROM

The Cochrane Library[6]

The *Cochrane Library* is an electronic library published four times a year and is the publishing arm of the Cochrane Collaboration. It contains four main elements. The first is the *Cochrane Database of Systematic Reviews* (CDSR). This is the main product of the Cochrane Collaboration and consists of systematic reviews that have been prepared by reviewers within specialist review groups. These reviews are published in full text with tables of the included trials and diagrammatic tables of meta-analyses. The reviews are maintained up to date as new evidence is published. To date approximately 1000 reviews of the effects of healthcare are available on the *Library*. The second part of this register is a large number of protocols that are essentially reviews in progress, with details of expected publication dates for the completed review.

The second main element is the *Cochrane Controlled Trials Register* (CENTRAL/CCTR). To carry out its task of 'preparing, maintaining and disseminating systematic reviews of the effects of healthcare', the Collaboration quickly realised that RCTs needed to be identified and brought together. This arose mainly because it became apparent that standard search methods using Medline and other databases did not identify all the RCTs. Many titles do not include the term 'randomised' or even 'trial', and only if the trial was tagged as a RCT when it was added to Medline can it be recovered as a RCT. The work of the collaboration has included a huge hand-search of the world's medical journals to identify RCTs. The fruit of this is published on the *Library* and also fed back to the US National Library of Medicine, the publishers of Medline, for the trials to be additionally tagged or added. There are currently over 270 000 RCTs on the *Cochrane Library* (2001, issue 1).

The York Database of Abstracts of Reviews of Effectiveness (DARE) is the third element and provides structured abstracts of good-quality systematic reviews gathered from the world literature and summarised by reviewers at the NHS Centre for Reviews and Dissemination at the University of York. It also includes abstracted reports of health technology assessments from around the world and abstracts of reviews produced by the *American Journal of Physicians (ACP) Journal Club.*

One of the challenges around the science of evidence-based medicine has been to ensure that sound scientific methods are used in the review process. This has led to research on the methods themselves and much of this is available in the fourth element of the *Library*, the *Cochrane Review Methodology Database* (CRMD).

In addition, there are details of the Cochrane Collaboration and the *Handbook*, which is an electronic guide to methodology for systematic reviews and details on the review process. This Handbook is several hundred pages in length.

The *Library* is supported by a powerful search facility, which allows for searching at a variety of levels, including the option to search using MeSH terms. The search works through each of the registers and displays the results which can be printed if required. The *Cochrane Library* is now available for searching via the Internet. This facility is only available by means of subscription.

Best Evidence

Another recent development is 'Best Evidence', a CD-ROM containing the full text of two major secondary publication journals: *ACP Journal Club* and *Evidence-based Medicine*. These two journals scan some 90 journals worldwide and produce reviews with a structured abstract and commentary, which seeks to put the findings into a clinical perspective.

It is clear that a great deal of validated and valuable information is available without the need to purchase textbooks, simply by using the resources available on the Internet. While the information provided by this means requires assessment, these skills are part of the pharmacist's expertise. Careful use of web browser and search engine software, together with organised book-marking of sites, can facilitate the rapid supply of quality validated information.

References

1   Smith R (1991) Where is the wisdom? The poverty of medical evidence. *BMJ*. **303**: 798–9.

2   Mott S (1998) A single point for information on all medicines. *Pharmaceutical Times*. **Sept**: 24–8.

3   Eng TR, Maxfield A, Patrick K *et al*. (1998) Access to health information and support. A public highway or a private road? *JAMA*. **280**: 1371–5.

4   Chi-Lum BI, Lundberg GD, Silberg WM (1996) Physicians accessing the Internet, the PAI project. An educational initiative [Editorial]. *JAMA*. **275**: 1361–2.

5   Jadad AR, Gagliardi A (1998) Rating health information on the Internet. Navigating to knowledge or Babel? *JAMA*. **279**: 611–4.

6   *The Cochrane Library*. Update Software, Oxford. Updated quarterly.

CHAPTER SIX

Appraising the evidence

Gathering evidence is an important part of the process in any evidence-based approach to either pharmacy or medicine, and the basis for good evidence has been laid down in previous chapters. It is now important to put mechanisms in place so that the evidence can be assessed for quality. There is no guarantee of quality attached to a published systematic review and so a number of tools which help to assess the likely usefulness of the evidence uncovered are described. One method for assessing the RCT was described in Chapter 3. In this section, tools for other types of publication are presented as well as some discussion of the difficulties of assessing evidence around harm.

Defining research

Research is a process of enquiry that produces knowledge. In the context of a healthcare system such as the NHS, it has certain features which include:

- searching for new knowledge necessary to improve performance of healthcare delivery or improve health
- generating results that are generalisable, i.e. of value to others who face similar problems
- being designed around a clear, well-defined study protocol that has been followed
- subjecting the study protocol to peer review
- obtaining the approval of a relevant ethics committee where necessary

- having clearly defined arrangements for project management
- reporting findings in a way that subjects them to critical examination and also makes them accessible to all who could benefit from them. This normally involves publication in a peer-reviewed journal.

Box 6.1   Features of NHS R&D

- Searches for new knowledge
- Generates results that are generalisable
- Has a clear, well-defined study protocol
- Subjects the study protocol to peer review
- Has the approval of an ethics committee
- Has clearly defined project management
- Reports findings to all who could benefit from them

Observational and experimental research

There are two ways to test a hypothesis, either by observation or by experiment.

Observational research

In observational research, the researcher observes a population or group of patients or manipulates data about those patients. Such data may come from interviews or from existing data sets, for example prescription analysis data or registries for particular diseases such as cancer or infectious disease. Surveys and case-control studies are examples of observational research. A great deal of the research around pharmacy services is observational in style.

Experimental research

In experimental research, an intervention is performed as a result of planning by a researcher. The most powerful type of experimental study is the RCT, because the methods used eliminate a great deal of the observer bias found in observational studies.

Tables 6.1 and 6.2 show the suitability of different research methodologies for evaluating different types of interventions or outcomes.

Table 6.1 Suitability of various research methodologies to evaluate interventions[1]

	Type of research				
Intervention	Qualitative research	Case-control	Cohort	RCT	Systematic review
Diagnosis			✓	✓✓	✓✓✓
Treatment			✓	✓✓	✓✓✓
Screening				✓✓	✓✓✓
Managerial innovation	✓	✓	✓	✓✓	✓✓✓

Table 6.2 Suitability of various research methodologies to evaluate outcomes[1]

	Type of research					
Intervention	Qualitative research	Surveys	Case-control	Cohort	RCT	Systematic review
Effectiveness of an intervention					✓✓	✓✓✓
Effectiveness of health service delivery	✓	✓	✓	✓	✓✓	✓✓✓
Safety	✓	✓			✓✓	✓✓✓
Acceptability	✓	✓			✓✓	✓✓✓
Cost-effectiveness					✓✓	✓✓✓
Appropriateness	✓	✓				✓✓✓
Quality	✓	✓	✓	✓		✓✓✓

Once evidence has been gathered, it is important that this information is then appraised or evaluated in some way. Most evidence contains some clues as to its value and these clues can help to determine the overall usefulness. Probably the most important question to ask is: 'Does the article address an issue of relevance to my practice?' If the answer is 'no', then move on to the next article. The whole point of appraisal is to determine how reliable that evidence is and to identify any flaws and bias likely to affect the outcome. Many articles are written to prove a theory or point and it is not difficult to find publications where the conclusions bear little relevance to the results actually described.

There are a number of check lists that help to evaluate published literature. A number of these have originated from the Critical Appraisal Skills Programme (CASP) in Oxford.[2]

Systematic reviews and overviews

The ten questions in Box 6.2 are extremely useful in appraising a systematic review. They are designed to be used as an aid to assist in the general reading of reviews as they now regularly appear in the mainline medical journals, but are also of use in assessing the value of a review for a specific inquiry. Reviews that score highly are likely to be valuable in practice.

Box 6.2   Check list for appraising a systematic review

Are the results of the review valid?

1   Did the review address a clearly focused issue?
    HINT: Is there a clear question being asked? Is it focused in terms of population and outcome?

2   Did the authors select the right sort of studies for the review?
    HINT: Did they look for randomised controlled trials? Other studies relevant to the question?

If the answer to the first two questions is 'no', there is little point in reading further.

3   Do you think the important, relevant studies were included?
    HINT: What databases were used? Were reference lists followed up? Was any attempt made to find unpublished data? Was there any attempt to find non-English studies?

4   Did the review's authors do enough to assess the quality of the included studies?

HINT: Was any assessment or scoring system applied to the papers?

5 If the results of the study have been combined, was it reasonable to do so?
   HINT: Are all the results clearly displayed? Are the results from different studies similar? Are reasons for variations in results discussed?

What are the results?

6 What is the overall result of the review?
   HINT: Is the overall result clearly expressed? Is the result expressed in some clear numerical expression, e.g. NNT, odds ratio?

7 How precise are the results?
   HINT: Are the confidence intervals expressed?

Will the results help locally?

8 Can the results be applied to the local population?
   HINT: Is there sufficient difference between the study population and the local environment to cause concern?

9 Were all clinically important outcomes considered?

10 Are the benefits worth the harms and costs?

Questions adapted from Oxman AD *et al.* (1994) Users' guides to the medical literature. VI. How to use an overview. *JAMA.* **272**(17): 1367–71.

Therapy and prevention studies

The series of questions in Box 6.3 develops further the concepts used in the scoring system for RCTs described in Chapter 3 (Table 3.1).

Box 6.3 Check list for appraising RCTs

Screening questions
1 Did the trial address a clearly focused issue?
2 Was the assignment of patients to treatments randomised?

3 Were all the patients who entered the trial properly accounted for at its conclusion?
   − was follow-up complete?
   − were patients analysed in the groups to which they were randomised?
4 Were patients, health workers and study personnel 'blind' to treatment?
5 Were the groups similar at the start of the trial?
6 Aside from the experimental intervention, were the groups treated equally?

What are the results?
7 How large was the treatment effect?
8 How precise was the estimate of the treatment effect?

Will the results help locally?
9 Can the results be applied to the local population?
10 Were all clinically important outcomes considered?
11 Are the benefits worth the harms and costs?

Questions adapted from Guyatt GH, Sackett DL, Cook DJ (1993) Users' guides to the medical literature. II. How to use an article about therapy or prevention. *JAMA.* **270**: 2598–601, **271**: 59–63.

Economic analyses

Economic analyses are being demanded yet can be very difficult to interpret. Often the arguments lack credibility or relate to meaningless financial concepts. The set of questions in Box 6.4 goes some way to enable some appraisal to be made.

Box 6.4   Check list for appraising economic evaluations

1 Was a well-defined question posed in an answerable form?
2 Was a comprehensive description of the competing alternatives given (i.e. can you tell who did what to whom, where and how often)? How were consequences and costs assessed and compared?
3 Was there evidence that the programme's effectiveness had been established?

4 Were all important and relevant consequences and costs for each alternative identified?
5 Were consequences and costs measured accurately in appropriate units (e.g. hours of nursing time, number of physician visits, years-of-life gained) prior to valuation?
6 Were consequences and costs valued credibly?
7 Were consequences and costs adjusted for differential timings (discounting)?
8 Was an incremental analysis of the consequences and costs of alternatives performed?
9 Was a sensitivity analysis performed? Will the results help in purchasing for local people?
10 Did the presentation and discussion of the results include all of the issues that are of concern to purchasers?
11 Were the conclusions of the evaluation justified by the evidence presented?
12 Can the results be applied to the local population?

Questions adapted from Drummond M, Stoddart GL, Torrance GW (1987) *Methods for the Economic Evaluation of Health Care Programmes*. Oxford University Press, Oxford.

Clinical guidelines

Guidelines are enjoying popularity, yet are often not evidence-based. The guide in Box 6.5 is useful both to the potential users of guidelines and also to those who write guidelines.

Box 6.5   Check list for appraising clinical guidelines

Are the recommendations valid?

Primary guides
1 Were the options for management and the projected outcomes of care clearly specified?
2 Was an explicit and sensible process used to identify, select and combine evidence?

Secondary guides
3 Was an explicit and sensible process used to consider the relative values of different outcomes associated with alternative practices?

4 Was the guideline subjected to a credible external review process?

5 Is the guideline likely to account for important recent developments?

What are the recommendations?

6 Are clear recommendations made?

7 Are important caveats identified?

Will the recommendations help you in caring for your patients?

8 Is the primary objective of the guideline consistent with your objective?

9 Are the recommendations applicable to your patients?

10 Are the expected benefits of guideline implementaiton worth the anticipated harms and costs?

Questions are adapted from Hayward RSA *et al.* (1995) Users' guides to the medical literature. VIII. How to use clinical practice guidelines. A. Are the recommendations valid? B. What are the results and will they help me in caring for my patients? *JAMA.* **274**(7): 570–4, 1630–2.

How to teach critical appraisal skills to trainees

These skills are fundamental to pharmacists but are rarely taught during basic training, although they are beginning to appear in some pre-registration training programmes. It is key that pharmacists acquire the skills required to critically appraise the literature in each of the following areas:

- therapy
- screening programmes
- treatment guidelines
- systematic reviews
- randomised controlled trials
- case-control studies
- cohort studies.

Assessing harm

It is important to have mechanisms in place to assess harmful effects so that treatments that do more harm than good can be identified. Experience of writing systematic reviews around pain interventions has shown that while RCTs are excellent evidence for effect, they are not so good at revealing adverse or unwanted effects. If a study is looking at the effects of a single dose of a particular treatment, it is not surprising that adverse events occur less frequently than in a chronic dosing regimen. In the UK, there is a reporting system for adverse events which encourages the completion of a record by clinicians or pharmacists. The information is then submitted to a central database. This system, one of many in the developed world, suffers from huge under-reporting and so the true picture is difficult to obtain.

Many estimates of the size of the problem have been published, usually quoting figures of 15–20% of hospitalised patients experiencing an adverse drug reaction (ADR). Ideally a meta-analysis of the literature around adverse drug reaction reporting is needed and fortunately one has been recently published by Lazarou et al.[3] This group used a WHO definition[4] of an ADR as:

> any noxious, unintended, and undesired effect of a drug, which occurs at doses used in humans for prophylaxis, diagnosis, or therapy.

This definition excludes therapeutic failures, intentional and accidental poisoning and drug abuse. It also excludes adverse events due to errors in drug administration or non-compliance. The group argued that such a conservative definition would help to avoid overestimating the incidence of ADRs.

Lazarou and his colleagues carried out a literature search across a good range of databases and described a set of criteria for inclusion of the studies. Sadly, they decided to consider only studies performed in the US. The literature search resulted in 153 studies, of which 39 were included in the meta-analysis. They used various outcome measures, which included numbers of ADRs and also two subsets: ADRin, for an ADR occurring to a patient while in hospital; and ADRad, for an ADR causing admission to hospital.

The overall incidence of serious ADRs was 6.7% (CI 5.2–8.2%) and of fatal ADRs 0.32% (0.23–0.41%). The authors reported that in 1994, over 2.2 million inpatients experienced serious ADRs and over 100 000 suffered fatal ADRs. This makes ADRs around the sixth leading cause of death in the USA (Box 6.6). When the data are analysed by ADRin and ADRad, the figures for death are 63 000 and 43 000 deaths respectively.

Box 6.6 Leading causes of death in US

Heart disease
Cancer
Stroke
Pulmonary disease
Accidents
Adverse drug reactions
Pneumonia
Diabetes

These figures, although based entirely on the North American experience, have clear implications for pharmacists wherever they practise. It is time that the issue of ADRs was moved higher up the clinical pharmacists' agenda.

The term 'iatrogenic disease' has been in use for over 40 years now, defined as:

> a disease that is independent of underlying disease and results from either the drug administration, medical or surgical acts for prophylaxis, diagnosis or other therapy.[8]

The actual size of problems associated with medicine use is probably unknown. This subject is termed drug misadventuring by some[6] and includes:

- an inherent risk when drug therapy is indicated
- a situation created by action or lack of action by the administration of a drug or drugs through which a patient is harmed, with effects ranging from mild discomfort to fatality
- an ability to generate an outcome which may or may not be related to pre-existing pathology or disease
- a possible attribution to human error or immunological response or idiosyncratic response
- an unexpected reaction which is therefore unacceptable to patient and practitioner.

A paper published in *JAMA*[3] in 1975 suggested that a radical rethink was needed around the whole issue of drug reactions. These included:

- methods to assign blame to a drug for an untoward effect
- a need to identify some baseline data for control groups
- some stratification by population and some measure of benefits to compare with the risks.

An overview of the ADR literature reveals some clear and interesting messages that should improve the management of this problem. The majority of ADRs are predictable. For example, if anticoagulants are used then some patients will bleed. Other useful pointers are: age, generally those over 60 years suffer more problems; gender, women tend to experience a slightly higher proportion of ADRs than men do; and number of prescription medications, with the problem getting worse for patients on five or more medicines.

Decision tree analysis

Decision tree analysis is a method of plotting out potential and real solutions to problems of a complex nature. It has found application in a wide variety of areas, including projecting sales of new merchandise, calculating risk strategies and in healthcare problems.

Ofman[8] and colleagues used this approach to outline management strategies for treating patients presenting with dyspepsia who were also seropositive for *Helicobacter pylori*. They showed that therapy costs of anti-*H.pylori* treatment saved approximately $500 per patient treatment and reduced the demand for endoscopy by over 50%.

An investigation[9] into screening for carotid stenosis reveals the options outlined in Figure 6.1. Evidence is then used to calculate the complication rates or any other data to populate the diagram. The authors of this study used RCT evidence as a starting point for their arguments and were able to show that screening in asymptomatic patients would lead to costs of over $120 000 per QALY. They argued correctly that this is not cost-effective. This study is

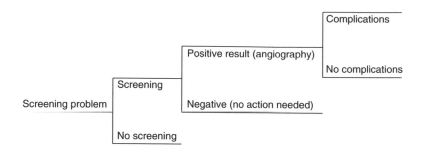

Figure 6.1: Decision tree analysis to calculate management strategy for screening for carotid stenosis.

not simply about costs but also about stopping interventions that are of limited benefit.

Decision tree analyses do rely on a number of assumptions which should be made explicit in the text. They can then be a useful means of bringing together a wealth of evidence and arriving at some definitive conclusions.

References

1 Gray JAM (1997) *Evidence-based Health Care: how to make health policy and management decisions*. Churchill Livingston, Glasgow.

2 CASP, Critical Appraisal Skills Programme [Web page]. Available at www. ihs.ox.ac.uk/casp/

3 Lazarou J, Pomeranz BH, Corey PN (1998) Incidence of adverse drug reactions in hospitalised patients. A meta-analysis of prospective studies. *JAMA.* **279**(15): 1200–5.

4 WHO (1966) *International Drug Monitoring; the role of the hospital*. Technical Report Series No 425. World Health Organisation, Geneva.

5 Smithells RW (1979) Iatrogenic hazards and their effects. *J Postgrad Med Educ.* **55**: 39–52.

6 Manesse HR (1989) Medication use in an imperfect world: drug misadventuring as an issue of public policy. *Am J Hosp Pharm.* **46**: 930.

7 Karch FE, Lasagna L (1975) Adverse drug reactions: a critical review. *JAMA.* **234**(12): 1236–41.

8   Ofman JJ, Etchason J, Fullerton S *et al.* (1997) Management strategies for *Helicobacter pylori*-seropositive patients with dyspepsia: clinical and economic consequences. *Ann Intern Med.* **126**: 280–91.

9   Lee TT, Soloman NA, Heidenreich PA *et al.* (1997) Cost effectiveness of screening for carotid stenosis in asymptomatic patients. *Ann Intern Med.* **126**: 337–46.

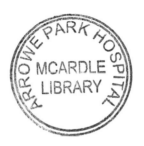

CHAPTER SEVEN

Getting the evidence into practice

In 1993, a project was launched in the Oxford region called GRiP: Getting research into practice (later known as GRiPP [and purchasing]). The concept was designed to bridge the gap between what was known as good evidence and what was actually happening in practice. Five topics were chosen (*see* Box 7.1), but more importantly, the project had an impact on the culture of the organisation.

Box 7.1   GRiPP topics

- The use of corticosteroids for women in pre-term labour
- The management of services to prevent and treat stroke
- The use of dilatation and curettage (D&C) for dysfunctional uterine bleeding in women under 40 years of age
- The use of grommets for children with glue ear
- Thrombolysis for people with acute MI

The GRiPP concept has much to offer those wishing to practise evidence-based pharmacy medicine management, covering important issues such as evaluating evidence for effectiveness of treatments and eliminating those treatments that are either of no value or, even worse, harmful. It could also be used to raise the profile around services that pharmacists regularly offer to the public, such as counselling on compliance, cessation of smoking or advice on minor ailments.

In addition, there are some key lessons for pharmacists who are regularly involved in writing guidelines. The main lessons are listed below.

- Carefully choose the topics
  - be explicit about the criteria and make sure they can be defended
  - consider how the main stakeholders will react to the choice of topic
  - involve the stakeholders from the beginning
  - do not rush into a choice of topic until full consideration has taken place.
- Consult with and involve local professions
  - ensure that the key players, both clinical and managerial, are involved right from the start
  - ensure there is frequent and meaningful communication, including discussion on the topic chosen (what and why), the nature of the evidence and the expected outcomes
  - keep groups small enough to be productive while keeping others informed of the process.
- Review the evidence
  - maintain a balance between the strength of the evidence and the effort put into the other elements of the process
  - involve practitioners in the whole process of evidence review to enhance the validity and credibility of the project
  - consider using locally produced evidence if it is available, but ensure it undergoes adequate peer review.
- Gather baseline data
  - decide early in the process what data should be collected so that changes can be measured when the project is launched
  - plan the data collection process carefully
  - do not let data collection become an end in itself.
- Develop evidence-based guidelines
  - if you are writing guidelines, look at the evidence around guideline use and implementation
  - do not try and import someone else's guidelines; however good they may be, these need to be adapted and adopted locally
  - guidelines developed in a suitable multidisciplinary forum are usually more effective

- ensure that guidelines are based on current best evidence and are not just a justification of current practice
- tackle areas of clinical importance and not just areas where there is strong evidence.
- Get the message out
  - plan the dissemination strategy carefully and review it regularly
  - make sure the findings are presented in a user-friendly way
  - think about the packaging. It should not be shabbily produced but equally should not be too glossy, either
  - consider getting the message out to patients and consumers early on in the process so there is local awareness of the developments
  - try and use channels of communication that already exist.
- Evaluate the results
  - carefully plan an evaluation into the process; this area is often neglected and leads to the downfall of otherwise worthy projects
  - in this evaluation, take note of:
    (i)   the scientific rigour of the evidence and guidelines
    (ii) the outcomes in terms of changed clinical behaviour and health status
    (iii) the organisational and political effects of the project
  - keep the evaluation simple and achievable
  - involve the key participants in the evaluation process.

The principles outlined above are readily transferable into a number of pharmacy projects. They could, for example, be used to develop community pharmacy services on health promotion or patient counselling. They are equally applicable in secondary care where significant formulary changes are being implemented or drug use evaluation is being undertaken.

Examples of evidence

Health promotion: stopping smoking

The development of health action zones (HAZs) in the UK has focused attention on improving public health and in particular has put the spotlight on the health risks of smoking.

The human costs of using tobacco have been well described by Robert Schrier and his colleagues from Colorado,[1,2] prompted by a levelling off in the prevalence of smoking in the US, at 26%, after two decades of decline. Their two reviews, containing 114 references mainly to the US literature, chart the health and economic costs.

Most people, especially health professionals, think they know the risks associated with tobacco smoking. Reading the first of these articles[1] and the report on mortality of British doctors,[3] is likely to make all except the most expert think again.

The way in which tobacco use constitutes the single largest threat to the health of the nation has been consistently understated – the more studies there are performed, the greater the number of diseases where tobacco use is reported to have an impact.

If cigarettes cost more, then fewer people will smoke them, especially women and members of the lowest socioeconomic groups where smoking prevalence is still as high as 50%.[4] Reduce prices, as happened in the UK between 1977 and 1979, and smoking goes up; increase prices, as has generally been the case since the early 1980s, and smoking falls. The commitment of Government to steadily increase the tax on cigarettes year by year should have an impact. UK Government initiatives are planning to build on this, with active targeting of smokers and provision of nicotine patches.

The economic cost of a cigarette

In the US, it has been estimated that the average lifetime medical costs for a smoker are $6000 greater than those for a non-smoker. The Congressional Office of Technology Assessment has estimated that the total financial cost of smoking to society in 1990 was $2.59 per pack of cigarettes (about £1.60 per packet at early-1999 exchange rates). There are numerous ways in which the economic costs of smoking and smoking-related diseases can be calculated, but whichever way they are calculated, all the numbers are big.

Other big numbers are seen in tobacco company profits – Philip Morris made more money in 1992 than any other US industrial corporation ($4900 million). (Ironically, some tobacco companies have diversified into insurance, which have higher charges for smokers than for non-smokers.) Another large number is that of tobacco company spending on advertising – $2000m a year by Philip Morris alone.

Tobacco advertising

When TV advertising of cigarettes was stopped in the US, the advertising revenue of magazines went up by an average of $5.5m a year, and smoking actually increased.

Buying sponsorship for sport is also very effective. For example, during the 1989 broadcast of the Marlboro Grand Prix, lasting 93 minutes, the Marlboro name was mentioned 11 times and the logo shown a staggering 5922 times. It had a total of 46 minutes of exposure, of which 18 minutes was 'clear, in-focus air time'.

Campaigns to prevent tobacco use

The second of the *New England Journal of Medicine* articles[2] has a plethora of interesting facts on economics, advertising and issues relating to preventing tobacco use. Although these are directed at the US, most issues relating to reducing tobacco use are relevant, including:

- increased taxation
- comprehensive smoking bans
- advertising and sponsorship bans
- restricting sales to children
- financial support for counter-advertising
- community education programmes.

All of these issues are important parts of strategies to prevent smoking in populations. What about the individual smoker – what can be offered by healthcare professionals to help in giving up smoking, and what is effective?

Nicotine replacement therapy

Nicotine replacement therapy (NRT) is based on the idea that replacing nicotine in the body allows smoking behaviour to be stopped. A gradual weaning of the subject from nicotine follows, without the pharmacological sequelae.

There have been three meta-analyses of NRT published recently, looking mainly at nicotine chewing gum and nicotine patches.[5-7] Although slightly different in the range of studies included and methods used, they all had the same conclusion that NRT is significant in helping smokers stop smoking.

Tang et al.[5] analysed 28 randomised trials of 2 mg nicotine gum, six trials of 4 mg nicotine gum and six trials of transdermal patch. They used as a main outcome measure the difference between per cent of control and NRT-treated patients who had stopped smoking at one year. The results showed that 2 mg nicotine chewing gum helped an extra 6% of smokers quit over controls, but this was as high as 11% in self-referred subjects and as low as 3% in invited subjects, suggesting that the desire to quit was essential.

When examined by dependency and whether patients were self-referred or invited, the results showed that nicotine gum was helpful in highly dependent subjects.

The meta-analysis by Silagy et al.[7] examined 53 trials, 42 with gum, nine with patch, one with intranasal spray and one with inhaler. The results were generally similar, although expressed differently. The odds ratios for abstinence were increased with use of NRT, but differently for different forms. This report also looked at the NNT to obtain one extra non-smoker at 12 months, beyond the number who would achieve that with the control intervention.

The nicotine patch was the particular focus of the third meta-analysis.[6] Here 17 studies were identified, with nearly 5100 subjects. At six months, 22% treated with patch had stopped smoking compared with 9% for placebo. The patch type (24 h versus 16 h), patch treatment duration (more or less than eight weeks), weaning, counselling format and intensity made no difference to the results. There was some evidence that intensive behavioural counselling had a modest effect on increasing rates of smoking cessation.

Unaided smoking cessation

What about all the smokers who give up on their own, without medical help; how do they do it? Lennox and Taylor[8] used postal questionnaires to investigate this in Aberdeen. The simple finding was that light and heavy smokers found it easier to give up than did moderate smokers.

Those who succeeded thought they had social support, and were more likely to have 'simply just stopped'. They were less likely to have used nicotine gum or to believe that smoking was harmful. Failures experienced more withdrawal symptoms and were likely to be tempted by other people smoking. Eleven per cent had never tried to stop; these were older, but were more likely to stop for financial reasons.

Behaviour therapy

A German report[9] of an RCT of structured extensive behaviour therapy compared with a single unstructured anti-smoking advice session given by a physician in diabetic patients, was disappointingly negative. Of 794 insulin-treated patients, only 89 consented to enter the study, in which smoking cessation was measured objectively by urinary cotinine.

After six months, 2/44 patients randomised to the intensive behaviour therapy had stopped, compared with 7/45 who received the unstructured intervention.

Smoking cessation in pregnancy

Because maternal smoking is associated with increased foetal risk and low birth weight, trying to prevent pregnant women smoking has top priority. One RCT[10] compared an immediate 20-minute intervention by a practice nurse with a two-hour evening class providing guidance on a self-help programme. Smoking cessation was confirmed by urinary cotinine measurement.

None of the women randomised to the intensive evening class attended, compared with 93% assigned to the immediate intervention. Rates of smoking cessation immediately after intervention, at 36 weeks gestation and post-partum, were about 6% for the 20-minute group and 14% for the evening class.

However, there is one study that shows some success. Again, this was an RCT begun in early pregnancy, with randomisation between standard obstetric care and an intervention with additional self-help materials on smoking cessation.[11]

Self-reported smoking behaviour was confirmed with a urinary cotinine test. This showed that 25% of women who said they were not smoking actually did smoke. The smoking cessation rates were not significantly different during pregnancy, at about 24%, but at eight weeks post-partum 29% of smokers had given up in the intervention group compared with under 10% in the non-intervention group. The cost of the intervention (self-help manual and audio-tapes) was $50–111 per patient.

Nicotine addiction through cigarette smoking is recognised as the largest single cause of poor health in the UK. NRT has clearly been demonstrated to help people give up smoking, and directed government policies on issues like tax are also of great value in deterring smokers.

Evidence around adverse effects

Adverse drugs and driving

Pharmacists regularly give patients advice about driving, in the form of a warning label, but what evidence is there that prescription drugs can impair fitness to drive? One study of deaths in road traffic accidents found tricyclic antidepressants in body fluids of 0.2% of victims, compared with alcohol (35%) or other drugs likely to affect the central nervous system (CNS) (7.4%).[12]

Morphine and driving

Reassuring results have come from a Finnish study of driving ability in cancer patients taking long-term morphine.[13] Although morphine given as a single dose to a healthy volunteer impairs reaction time, co-ordination, attention and memory, this is not true for patients on long-term stable doses.

The authors used a battery of tests designed for professional drivers (Austrian Road Safety Board, as used for Helsinki bus drivers) to compare the performance of 24 patients on continuous morphine (mean 210 mg oral morphine daily) with that of 25 pain-free patients who took no regular analgesics. The morphine patients had been on a stable dose (twice daily sustained-release formulation) for at least two weeks.

There was no significant difference between the morphine patients and the controls on the driving simulator tests. Balancing ability with eyes closed was significantly worse with morphine, finger-tapping with preferred hand was better. The conclusion was that patients on long-term stable dosing with morphine should be at no greater risk to themselves or to other road users.

Changing the dose

How long should drivers taking morphine stay off the road after changing dose? Perhaps the best information comes from a study[14] which suggested that an increase in the dose by 30% will impair cognitive function for one week after the increase. The study indicated that at least the first three to five days may be 'impaired'. It might be safe to use this time limit in the absence of more conclusive evidence.

NSAID-induced gastrointestinal injury

NSAIDs are among the most effective analgesics for both acute and chronic pain (*see* Figure 4.2). They are, however, associated with a number of adverse effects, which are generally well known, the most important being the effect on gastrointestinal (GI) mucosa. What is generally not appreciated is the frequency with which these side effects occur. There are other important side effects, such as the effect on the kidney and also on asthma, but this section will concentrate on evidence for serious GI adverse effects. Reliable evidence for adverse events is difficult to find; adverse event reporting schemes suffer from serious under-reporting and RCTs are not a reliable way to collect data on adverse effects as the numbers of participants are rarely high enough. NSAID-related GI problems are serious, as minor GI discomfort can lead to ulceration and in some cases the ulcers bleed. Some of these bleeds can be fatal. Three large-scale surveys give an insight into this problem.

The first, from Rotherham and Stockport in England,[15] carried out a retrospective case-control study in two large general hospitals. Blower *et al.* looked at all the emergency admissions for upper GI disease in these two hospitals. Matched controls were identified from other emergency admissions. There were 620 emergencies in a one-year period (1990–91). The main presentation was haemorrhage (59%). Blood transfusion was required in 36% of all cases, and in 50% of those taking NSAIDs. Overall mortality was 20% in NSAID users compared with 14% in those not taking these drugs.

These data can be extrapolated for a population group of one million and the data are shown in Table 7.1.

Table 7.1 Retrospective case-control study of emergency admissions for upper GI disease

Age range (years)	% of population	Number	% NSAID prescriptions	No. of prescribed NSAIDs	Annual no. of admissions for one million population
16–45	42	420 000	5	21 000	10
45–64	19	190 000	17	32 300	50
65–74	12	120 000	19	22 800	40
> 75	7	70 000	22	15 400	140
			Total		240

In the second study, Hawkey et al.[16] interviewed 500 patients aged over 60 who were admitted with peptic ulcer bleeds to two hospitals in Nottingham over a five-year period. They then looked at the general practice prescribing of NSAIDs for the patients interviewed. They were able to show that NSAID prescribing was the major factor in determining emergency admissions in this group and demonstrated a wide range in prescribing rates for NSAIDs, from 137 items per 1000 population to 833 items per 1000 population. The Blower data showed rates of around 200 prescriptions per 1000 population. The average admission rate was 15 per 100 000 population or approximately one episode of a bleeding ulcer for every 3000 prescriptions of an NSAID in the over-60 age group.

A cohort study from Scotland[17] is the third in the series on NSAID risks. This group looked at the over-50-year-old population ($N = 52\,000$) who received at least one prescription for an NSAID and were admitted to hospital with a GI event over a three-year period. There was a control group of 72 000. They found that approximately 2% of those who had received an NSAID were admitted, compared to 1.4% of controls.

The place of gastric protection for oral NSAIDs

A number of clinical papers[18,19] have looked at the risk factors, which are listed in Box 7.2. While there is a strong argument for protection for all patients on chronic NSAIDs, these risk factors require particular attention.

Box 7.2   Risk factors for NSAID-induced gastric problems

- Age of 75 years or more
- History of peptic ulcer
- History of GI bleeding
- History of heart disease

The same papers also give some indication of the best treatments for NSAID-induced GI problems and enable NNTs to be calculated. The first[18] is a systematic review of 24 reports covering 4325 patients. Misoprostol significantly reduced the rate of gastric ulcers in both the short term – between one and two weeks (NNT 8) – and long term – > four weeks (NNT 12). The H_2 antagonists did not reduce the rate of gastric ulcers in either the short- or long-term trials. Several RCTs give NNTs for ulcer prevention with NSAID use, as follows:

- omeprazole 20 mg, NNT 3
- misoprostol 800 micrograms, NNT 6.[20]

Evidence of treatment

Evidence of poor effect

Does TENS work?

TENS (transcutaneous electronic nerve stimulation) is a popular method of pain relief offered by physiotherapists and others for chronic pain, and by midwives for the pain associated with labour. The weekend newspapers often contain adverts for TENS devices.

According to a Canadian technology assessment paper,[21] TENS appears to be widely used across Canada. The authors surveyed 50 hospitals with 200 or more beds, and estimated that there were over 450 000 uses of TENS in Canadian hospitals each year with widespread use in physiotherapy, for acute pain (used by 93% of hospitals), for labour and delivery (43%), and for chronic pain (96%).

TENS in acute pain

The Canadian study[21] included randomised and non-randomised studies, although it split them for descriptive analysis. They reviewed 39 studies (34 randomised, 5 not randomised) of postoperative pain, dental pain, dysmenorrhoea and cervical pain. They describe the results as varied, but it is hard to find much that is good about TENS. The review suggested that of the 34 original papers that reported the results of randomised studies, 19 reached positive conclusions about TENS, while the other 15 reached a negative or balanced conclusion.

Table 7.2   TENS in postoperative pain

	Analgesic result	
	Positive	*Negative*
Randomised	2	15
Inadequate or not randomised	17	2

In a review limited to randomised studies in acute postoperative pain,[22] TENS was judged by the reviewers to be no better than placebo in 15 out of 17 studies (Table 7.2). Of 19 trials with pain outcomes that were not randomised, the authors of 17 of the 19 original papers had concluded that TENS had a beneficial effect. This is another good example of bias in non-randomised studies.

TENS in labour pain

The Canadian review[21] summarised six of nine randomised trials as reaching negative conclusions. This is a similar result to that of a second review[23] that examined eight reports, of which five were judged to have a negative result, with TENS no better than placebo or sham-TENS. However, the three studies that were judged to be positive were positive only on weak outcomes such as additional pain-relieving measures and increased time to epidural local anaesthetic.

Additional analgesic interventions were significantly less likely with the use of TENS,[23] with a NNT of 14 (95% CI 7–119) for one woman in labour to be spared an epidural or intramuscular injection. Of the four trials that reported this outcome, only the two smaller trials (23 women receiving TENS) were statistically significant, while the two larger studies (208 women receiving TENS) were not significantly different from placebo.

A randomised trial of 94 women in the first stage of labour published since the reviews were done[24] undermines even this possible level of benefit. It found no difference in analgesic requirement between active TENS and disabled TENS equipment, nor any difference on pain scores.

TENS in chronic pain

The Canadian review[21] found 20 randomised trials, of which nine were definitely positive for TENS on some measure, while eight were negative for TENS.

A disappointing review limited to chronic low back pain[25] included just six papers. Two of the original studies were of electroacupuncture, which is not the same as TENS. One trial had only ten patients randomised, six to TENS and four to placebo. TENS was not significantly different from placebo. Electroacupuncture was significantly better than placebo, but in only two studies with 30 patients given electroacupuncture.

Comment

First, there are methodological considerations. Adequate blinding of TENS is extremely difficult, so that most trials should at best be regarded as open, even if described as blinded. This must confer some degree of bias towards TENS.

Second, there was a tendency in all these reviews to point to an overall lack of methodological rigour in the original studies (while acknowledging that these trials are difficult). The trials with the best methods tended to produce negative results.

Then there is the issue of statistical validity. Many of these trials make a number of different measurements, only some of which show statistical benefit. So choosing just those measurements which are significant, and ignoring those that are not significant, can give a spurious weight to a review. This is especially true when statistical benefit is of dubious clinical value. So any reading of these reviews should be sceptical, especially when, as in acute postoperative pain, there are adequate alternatives. For labour pain, there may be an argument for good-quality trials which examine the issue of delay or avoidance of interventions such as epidurals or intramuscular opiates, which carry some risk to mother or baby.

Chronic pain is a different matter. Where the evidence is not clear-cut, where some patients are seen to benefit and where alternatives may not work for all patients, then carrying on using TENS until there is some clarification makes sense. That does put some pressure on getting well-designed studies of sufficient power to provide practically useful answers under way.

Some evidence of effect

Antibiotics for acute otitis media

Ear infections in children are common. Despite there being over 170 published clinical trials, there is no consensus on the best drug for the initial therapy for acute otitis media (AOM).

Meta-analysis

A meta-analysis of 35 randomised studies involving antimicrobial drugs in 5400 children may help. This very detailed study[26] is a great example of how systematic reviews can be done; the authors started with a written protocol defining the methods and objectives of the meta-analysis.

Study inclusion

To be included, studies had to be RCTs of antimicrobial drugs for the initial empirical treatment of simple AOM. The authors give exact definitions of what they mean for each of these phrases to avoid any doubt:

- Simple AOM – new or recurrent episodes of AOM in patients without underlying disorders.
- AOM – bulging or opacification of the tympanic membrane with or without reddening, with symptoms of acute infection.
- Initial empirical therapy – treatment of new-onset AOM without knowledge of the specific causative agent.
- Therapeutic antimicrobial agents – drugs administered to treat established AOM – with individual drugs defined.

- Randomised controlled studies – allocation of subjects by chance to one or more concurrent treatment groups, at least one of them involving a study drug as defined.

Their initial searching strategy identified 286 studies. The progression from that to the final tally of 30 is set out with the reasons for each exclusion given.

Outcome measures

The primary end point was the clinical response to antimicrobial therapy. This was defined as the absence of all presenting signs and symptoms of AOM at the evaluation point closest to 7–14 days after therapy started. The appearance of the tympanic membrane, if reported, should be improved.

Neither middle-ear effusion nor the lack of a bacteriological cure was grounds for considering a specific treatment a failure. All outcomes less than successful as defined, including unilateral resolution of bilateral AOM, were considered primary end point failures. Patients, rather than ears, were the unit of analysis.

Results

Sixty nine study arms were identified in the 30 trials. The results are shown in Table 7.3. Pre-treatment tympanocentesis increased the primary control rates by 6.5% (95% CI 3–10%).

This paper has many different comparisons between different drugs and a number of sensitivity analyses. The main findings of effect were the comparisons of penicillin or any antimicrobial agent against placebo or no drug controls. Antibiotics were clearly

Table 7.3   Results of meta-analysis of RCTs of antimicrobial drugs for the treatment of AOM

Intervention	No. of study arms	Resolution of AOM
Controls	4	70% ± 17%
Standard-spectrum antibiotics	26	77% ± 17%
Extended-spectrum antibiotics	39	86% ± 13%

better than controls (no antibiotic) but no one antibiotic was shown to be superior to any other.

Number-needed-to-treat

The NNT was calculated in the paper as 7. Six of every seven children with AOM either do not need antibiotics for primary control or will not respond to antibiotic therapy. All seven children have to be treated because we cannot predict which one of the seven is both at risk for failure and responsive to antibiotics. This can also be stated as: for every seven children who present with AOM and receive an antibiotic, one will respond who would not have done so if they had not been treated.

Provided that the antibiotic given is safe, well-tolerated and affordable, this need to treat many to control a few would be offset by a 14% higher primary control rate and a potentially lower incidence of suppurative complications.

Conclusion

The authors give a qualified 'yes' to the question of whether antibiotics should be part of the initial empirical therapy for AOM in children. As always, there are qualifications, and these are carefully explained. As is so often the case, no single paper, or meta-analysis in this case, gives the entire result. But meta-analyses like this provide policy makers with the raw material from which to forge guidelines based on solid evidence.

Good evidence for effect

An overview of randomised trials from *JAMA*,[27] which gives more information than that published in the original trials, is a good example of the evidence available on statins.

The studies

The systematic review looked for randomised trials which involved:

- statin drugs alone used to reduce lipid levels, rather than multi-

factorial interventions including another type of cholesterol-lowering drug
- inclusion of data on deaths and/or strokes.

Sixteen studies were found. The researchers wrote to the authors of the original studies and consequently were able to give information on fatal and non-fatal strokes and MI not always given in the original reports. But some of the studies were small and short. The 13 studies which had over 100 patients in any treatment group and which were of at least six months' duration are included here; these data were originally reviewed in *Bandolier*.

Outcomes

There are many different outcomes (death from any cause, fatal and non-fatal strokes and MI, to name the most important). *Bandolier* brought all these together as 'anything bad', which consists of deaths from any cause, plus non-fatal stroke, plus non-fatal MI. This may seem a bit simplistic, but has the distinct advantage that it gives many events and can give an overall NNT for 'all bad things'.

Results

Primary prevention

Three trials examined statins for primary prevention, two using pravastatin and one lovastatin. They involved 7961 patients treated for an average of 4.6 years, and heavily weighted by the WOSCOPS trial. The NNTs are shown in Table 7.4.

Table 7.4 Statins in primary prevention (7961 patients, mean 4.6 years)

Event	NNT (95% CI)
All causes of death	107 (58 to 617)
All strokes	330 (123 to no benefit)
All coronary heart disease	48 (32 to 95)
All strokes plus all coronary heart disease	42 (28 to 80)
All deaths plus non-fatal strokes plus non-fatal MIs	35 (24 to 63)

The 'all bad things' NNT was 35 (24 to 63). This means that 35 people have to be treated with a statin for 4.6 years to prevent a bad thing (death, stroke or heart attack) happening in one of them.

Secondary prevention

Ten trials examined statins for secondary prevention, two using simvastatin, four pravastatin and four lovastatin. They involved 20 589 patients treated for an average of 2.9 years and were heavily weighted by the 4S, CARE and EXCEL trials. The NNTs are shown in Table 7.5.

Table 7.5   Statins in secondary prevention (20 589 patients, mean 2.9 years)

Event	NNT (95% CI)
All causes of death	33 (28 to 42)
All strokes	71 (55 to 98)
All coronary heart disease	14 (13 to 16)
All strokes plus all coronary heart disease	12 (11 to 14)
All deaths plus non-fatal strokes plus non-fatal MIs	11 (10 to 13)

The 'all bad things' NNT was 11 (10 to 13). This means that 11 people have to be treated with a statin for 2.9 years to prevent a bad thing (death, stroke or heart attack) happening in one of them.

Of course, this is a summation across all trials, with three different drugs, with different rates of events with controls, reflecting different populations and duration of the trials. It is

Table 7.6   Statins compared in secondary prevention

Statin	Number	Duration (years)	Total patient years	Events with controls (%)	NNT (95% CI)
Lovastatin	9250	1	9250	2	187 (86 to no benefit)
Pravastatin	6514	3.7	24 102	15	27 (19 to 51)
Simvastatin	4825	5.3	25 573	33	10 (9 to 15)

possible to do an analysis by drug, and this is presented in Table 7.6. However, direct comparison is not possible.

With lovastatin, although over 9000 people have been in trials, the trials were only for an average of one year, and with low numbers of events. So the NNT is high at 187.

With pravastatin, over 6500 people were involved, with trials going on for an average of nearly four years. The number of events with controls was 15% and the NNT was 27.

With simvastatin, just under 5000 people were studied for over five years. There was a large number of events with controls (33%), and the NNT was low at 10.

Adverse effects

The systematic review found no evidence for any increased risk in non-stroke mortality, nor any significant risk of cancer over control.

Comment

Many groups are seeking to produce guidance for clinicians on the use of statins. That guidance is best founded on solid evidence, and the best evidence comes from quality systematic reviews. There is an excellent example of using systematic reviews in practice guidelines by Cook et al.,[28] which is worth reading.

The evidence is conclusive: statins work, and work well. Key questions being asked include which patient and which statin? Many answers to these and other questions will be driven by cost influences. Perhaps they ought to be driven by the weight of evidence as well – evidence which will change as more studies report, and as other evidence from audit and elsewhere becomes available. When it does, and if it changes the picture, then guidance can change with it.

Cost-effectiveness

This always seems to be the downside of cholesterol lowering, whatever the intervention used. A systematic review of the cost-effectiveness literature is a good place to start looking for advice.[29]

The problem, as the authors tell us, is that while there is general agreement among the studies, there is high sensitivity to the assumptions used, especially in screening strategies. The major conclusions were:

- Cost-effectiveness of primary prevention with cholesterol-lowering drugs is extremely variable, depending on age at start of treatment and risk profile.
- Pharmacological intervention is least cost-effective in the young and the elderly.
- Cost-effectiveness improves when treatment is targeted at high-risk individuals.
- Statins are more cost-effective than other interventions at reducing cholesterol-related coronary events.

References

1   Bartecchi CE, MacKenzie TD, Schrier RE (1994) The human costs of tobacco use 1. *NEJM.* **330**: 907–12.

2   MacKenzie TD, Bartecchi CE, Schrier RE (1994) The human costs of tobacco use 2. *NEJM.* **330**: 975–80.

3   Doll R, Peto R, Wheatley K *et al.* (1994) Mortality in relation to smoking: 40 years' observation on male British doctors. *BMJ.* **309**: 901–10.

4   Townsend J, Roderick P, Cooper J (1994) Cigarette smoking by socio-economic group, sex and age: effects of price, income and health publicity. *BMJ.* **309**: 923–7.

5   Tang JL *et al.* (1994) How effective is nicotine replacement therapy in helping people to stop smoking? *BMJ.* **308**: 21–6.

6   Fiore MC, Smith SS, Jorenby DE, Baker DB (1994) The effectiveness of the nicotine patch for smoking cessation. *JAMA.* **271**: 1940–7.

7   Silagy C, Mant D, Fowler G, Lodge M (1994) Meta-analysis on efficacy of nicotine replacement therapies in smoking cessation. *Lancet.* **343**: 139–42.

8   Lennox AS, Taylor RJ (1994) Factors associated with outcome in unaided smoking cessation, and a comparison of those who have never tried to stop smoking with those who have. *Br J Gen Pract.* **44**: 245–50.

9   Sawicki PT, Didjurgeit D, Ÿhlhauser IM, Berger M (1993) Behaviour therapy versus doctor's anti-smoking advice in diabetic patients. *J Intern Med.* **234**: 407–9.

10 O'Connor AM, Davies BL, Dulberg CS *et al.* (1992) Effectiveness of a

pregnancy smoking cessation program. *J Obstet Gynecol Neonatal Nursing*. **21:** 385–92.

11 Petersen L, Handel J, Kotch J *et al.* (1992) Smoking reduction during pregnancy by a program of self-help and clinical support. *Obstet Gynecol*. **79:** 924–30.

12 Everest JT, Tunbridge RJ, Widdop B (1989) The incidence of drugs in road accident fatalities. Transport Research Laboratory, Crowthorne.

13 Vainio A, Ollila J, Matikainen E, Rosenberg P, Kalso E (1995) Driving ability in cancer patients receiving long-term morphine analgesia. *Lancet*. **346:** 667–70.

14 Bruera E, Macmillan K, Hanson J, MacDonald N (1989) The cognitive effects of the administration of narcotic analgesics in patients with cancer pain. *Pain*. **39:** 13–16.

15 Blower AI, Brooks A, Fenn CG *et al.* (1997) Emergency admissions for upper gastrointestinal disease and their relation to NSAID use. *Aliment Pharmacol Ther*. **11:** 283–91.

16 Hawkey CJ, Cullen DJ, Greenwood DC *et al.* (1997) Prescribing of nonsteroidal anti-inflammatory drugs in general practice: determinants and consequences. *Aliment Pharmacol Ther*. **11:** 293–8.

17 MacDonald TM, Morant SV, Robinson GC *et al.* (1997) Association of upper gastrointestinal toxicity of non-steroidal anti-inflammatory drugs with continued exposure: cohort study. *BMJ*. **315:** 1333–7.

18 Koch M, Dezi A, Ferrario F *et al.* (1996) Prevention of non-steroidal anti-inflammatory drug-induced gastrointestinal mucosal injury. *Arch Intern Med*. **156:** 2321–32.

19 Silverstein FE, Graham DY, Senior JR *et al.* (1995) Misoprostol reduces serious gastrointestinal complications in patients with rheumatoid arthritis receiving nonsteroidal anti-inflammatory drugs. *Ann Intern Med*. **123:** 241–9.

20 Hawkey CJ, Karrasch JA, Szczepanki L *et al.* (1998) Omeprazole compared with misoprostol for ulcers associated with nonsteroidal anti-inflammatory drugs. *NEJM*. **338:** 727–34.

21 Reeve J, Menon D, Corabian P (1996) Transcutaneous electrical nerve stimulation (TENS): a technology assessment. *International Journal of Technology Assessment*. **12**(2): 299–324.

22 Carroll D, Tramer M, McQuay H *et al.* (1996) Randomisation is important in studies with pain outcomes: systematic review of transcutaneous electrical nerve stimulation in acute postoperative pain. *Br J Anaesthesia*. **77:** 798–803.

23 Carroll D, Tramer M, McQuay H *et al.* (1997) Transcutaneous electrical nerve

stimulation in labour pain: a systematic review. *Br J Obstet Gynaecol.* **104**: 169–75.

24 van der Ploeg JM, Vervest HAM, Liem A (1996) Transcutaneous nerve stimulation (TENS) during the first stage of labour: a randomized clinical trial. *Pain.* **68**: 75–8.

25 Gadsby JG, Flowerdew MW (1999) The effectiveness of transcutaneous electrical nerve stimulation (TENS) and acupuncture-like transcutaneous electrical nerve stimulation (ALTENS) in the treatment of patients with chronic low back pain. In: *The Cochrane Library*. Update Software, Oxford.

26 Rosenfeld R, Vertrees JE, Carr J et al. (1994) Clinical efficacy of antimicrobial drugs for acute otitis media: meta-analysis of 5400 children from thirty-three randomised trials. *Journal of Pediatrics.* **124**: 355–67.

27 Hebert PR, Gaziano JM, Chan KS, Hennekens CH (1997) Cholesterol lowering with statin drugs, risk of stroke, and total mortality. *JAMA.* **278**: 313–21.

28 Cook DJ, Greengold NL, Ellrodt NL, Weingarten SR (1997) The relationship between systematic reviews and practice guidelines. *Ann Intern Med.* **127**: 210–16.

29 Morris S, McGuire A, Caro J, Pettitt D (1997) Strategies for the management of hypocholesterolaemia: a systematic review of the cost-effectiveness literature. *J Health Serv Res Policy.* **2**(4): 231–50.

Managing knowledge

For many practitioners, finding a way to store the vast amount of data they receive and to retrieve valuable information is quite a challenge. Information is usually acquired in two ways. First, there is the useful material that is collected in the course of work and squirreled away for future use; and second, there is the information gathered as part of specific projects or exercises.

There are many tried and tested filing systems for papers or research articles which enable storage into pre-determined categories that can expand or contract according to need. These are often linked to a computer file which can be used to log what exists. The disadvantages of such methods are that material is often difficult to retrieve and that every time a reference needs to be cited, it has to be retyped. Storing paper is relatively easy in the short term, but as the pile grows it becomes increasingly difficult to find that article you know you have somewhere. This is particularly a challenge for pharmacy drug information services that need to handle a great deal of paper efficiently.

One of the most useful tools is the bibliographic database, which has been popular in many research settings both within and outside medicine, but which has not penetrated the pharmacy world to any great extent.

> Unfortunately, unorganised growth, be it of body tissue or of references, usually ends in death.
> Alarçon[1]

An article by Brian Haynes and colleagues[2] published in 1986 asked some useful questions about need for storage and suggested some simple low-tech solutions. The questions included:

- How much time are you willing to put into maintaining the file?
- What library facilities do you have at hand and use regularly?
- How many functions do you need your personal file to support?
- Allowing for growth, how many articles is your file likely to hold?
- How often do you or will you use your file?
- How familiar are you with the contents of your file?
- How important is it for you to cross-reference articles?
- How much access do you have or will you have to computers?
- How simple or complex a solution is best suited to you?

The authors developed a scale from one to five for answering each question. One is for the simplest or lowest answers and five is for large, complex systems. There are useful hints on setting up files based on suggested headings and related to the complexity of the system required.

Personal bibliographic databases

Many of us have started with a crude physical filing system often made up of articles torn from journals, usually in a fairly random way. There comes a point where these systems take on the features of a black hole and what goes in rarely, if ever, comes out or can be found. Personal bibliographic databases are simply structured database files with some useful features which enable the black-hole problem to be eliminated even for very large filing systems.

The basic layout of the database is designed to handle information published in various formats, e.g. journal articles, books etc, and the fields are set up to hold that information. There are additional fields which include sections for key words and reference numbers. The simplest use of the database is to manually add information into the fields in a logical sequence. The data are held as records that can then be searched using a variety of options, such as author, date of publication, keywords, etc. It is then a simple task to assign a number to the record that matches a number added to the original article, e.g. in numerical order of collection, and subsequently to retrieve the hard copy of a reference by searching for key words, etc. Databases of many thousands of papers can be built up in this way and single articles identified in seconds. For example, a single reference in a ProCite database of 20 000 records can be found in less than five seconds.

There are some useful additions that make this type of software particularly valuable. First, searches that have been carried out electronically using a database such as Medline can be downloaded directly into the personal bibliographic database using a linking software package such as Bibliolinks. Translators are available for most of the commonly used databases and this facility enables a database of useful information to be created quickly without rekeying the information. The full record, including the abstract, is usually imported, thus extending the search possibilities within the personal database.

Second, all the software packages have the means for either simple or complex searches. In ProCite, the following options are available to search a database.

It is possible to build a search expression in the text box. You can type the text or use the fields, operators and terms buttons to help build your search expression. For example, you could enter:

AUTHOR = Smith and KEYWORDS = Asthma

It is possible to search by date or a range of dates. You can save your search expression with the expressions button, so you can perform the same search again after more records are entered. Or, you can save the list of records that results from your current search by highlighting them and using the group menu to save them to a group.

The third key feature is the ability to link a manuscript to the database to generate a reference list. This task, which is usually time-consuming and tedious, is quickly performed, as the word processing package commonly but not necessarily used, Word, interacts to find the references mentioned, marks the text in the appropriate way, e.g. by adding a superscript number, and produces the reference list. Various styles of reference are available, so if your manuscript that uses, for example, Vancouver style is rejected by your favourite journal, it can be submitted with ease to another journal which requires, say, Harvard formatting.

Box 8.1   Example from ProCite

Author Analytic (01): Carroll, D.// Jadad, A.// King, V.// Wiffen, P.// Glynn, C.// McQuay, H.

Article Title (04): Single-dose, randomised, double-blind, double-dummy cross-over comparison of extradural and i.v. clonidine in chronic pain

Journal Title (03): Br J Anaesth

Date of Publication (20): 1993

Volume Identification (22): 71

Issue Identification (24): 5

Page(s): 665–9

ISSN (4): 0007-0912

Notes (42): HC

Abstract (43): We studied 10 patients with chronic back pain who had claimed benefit with a previous extradural dose of clonidine 150 micrograms combined with local anaesthetic. We compared a single dose of clonidine 150 micrograms given by either the extradural or i.v. route in a double-blind, randomised, double-dummy and cross-over fashion, with 80% power to detect a difference in the analgesic effect of the two routes. Pain intensity, pain relief, adverse effects, mood, sedation and vital signs were assessed by a nurse observer. I.v. clonidine produced significantly ($P < 0.04$) greater analgesia than extradural clonidine in one of the five analgesic outcome measures. Clonidine given by either route produced statistically significant sedation and significant decreases in arterial pressure and heart rate. In this study, extradural clonidine had no significant clinical advantages compared with i.v. clonidine, clonidine 150 micrograms by either route produced a high incidence of adverse effects.

Keywords (45): Yes/Chronic non-malignant pain/Pharmacological intervention/Adult/Aged/Analgesia, Epidural/Clonidine administration and dosage/Clonidine adverse effects/Double Blind Method/Injections, Intravenous/Middle Age/Pain Measurement/Back Pain drug therapy/Clonidine therapeutic use/ Comparative Study/Female/Human/Male/Support, Non U.S. Gov't

The reference appears as follows when presented in Vancouver format:

1. Carroll D, Jadad A, King V, Wiffen P, Glynn C, McQuay H. Single-dose, randomised, double-blind, double-dummy cross-over comparison of extradural and i.v. clonidine in chronic pain. Br J Anaesth 1993; 71(5): 665-9.

It is beyond the scope of this book to recommend a particular package, but a number are available including Reference Manager, ProCite, Idealist and EndNote. Other less well-known packages include Papyrus, Citation 7 and I-Cite. Details of contact addresses and Websites for personal bibliographic databases are listed in Appendix 2. A review of three of these databases can be found on the Web (www.biblio-tech.com/html/pbms.html).

Developing a knowledge management strategy

In reality, practitioners need a strategy to cope with the volume and range of material available. It is easy to think of continuous professional development as the answer, but that only partly meets the need. Attending workshops or lectures may be interesting, but they may not be what we need.

Professor Sackett[3] in *Clinical Epidemiology: a basic science for clinical medicine* makes the following points.

- As soon as formal education is complete, we hit the 'slippery slope of declining clinical competence'.
- It is not what we don't know that gets us into trouble, it is what we do know but in reality is wrong.

- The rate of advance in medical literature is not an excuse; we only need to know a tiny part of it.
- We can wait for others to tell us what we need to know, but we will always lag behind.

What is the answer? Here are some points for consideration.

- Concentrate on the peer-reviewed literature that provides the best yield for your interest or speciality. This is quite difficult, as pharmacy is particularly poor at producing peer-reviewed material. However, parts of the *Pharmaceutical Journal* are refereed. It may mean you have to seek out some of the medical journals either in the library or on the Internet. (For a list of peer-reviewed pharmacy journals, *see* Appendix 1.)
- Read only original articles of clinical trials or systematic reviews that are likely to have an impact on your own practice.
- Scan the methods and results sections to ensure the article is likely to come up with a valid answer.
- Develop a reading habit.
- Collaborate with colleagues and share journals around.
- Develop a strategy and stick to it.

This sounds like time for action, so what might be included in a strategy?

- Determine which journals you should read on a regular basis by conducting a personal survey of what you currently read and what can be derived from this reading. Seriously consider deleting those journals which give low yield.
- Consider scanning index pages as a means of maintaining awareness of content.
- Add as many high-yield journals to your list as you can manage, and consider sharing journals with colleagues or other departments.
- Develop a library habit; avoid the trap of believing that keeping up to date is somehow not a part of the job.
- Set aside a limited amount of time for Internet browsing to stay aware of developments, new guidelines, etc.

Teaching knowledge management skills to others

Pharmacists need to be taught sets of basic skills to maintain a good level of ongoing professional development.

Searching

In an ideal world a pharmacist would use a local drug information unit or medical librarian. There are often situations where information is required quickly, and pharmacists should be competent to find evidence for themselves. The following minimum competencies should be acquired:

- the ability to identify appropriate sources of evidence to answer a particular query
- the ability to carry out a search of Medline without the help of a librarian and to find at least 60% of the reviews or research studies that would have been identified by an expert searcher
- the ability to construct simple search strategies on Medline using Boolean operators such as 'AND' and 'OR' (*see* Chapter 3) for:
  - the following healthcare terms:
    - treatment
    - test
  - the following service characteristics:
    - effectiveness
    - safety
    - acceptability
    - appropriateness
    - quality
    - cost-effectiveness
- the ability to download the end product into reference management software. It is appreciated that this goes beyond the current skills of many pharmacists and also of a good number who work in drug information units.

Unfortunately, skills tend to atrophy if not used, and therefore regular refresher sessions are required to ensure skills are maintained.

Scanning

All pharmacists should seek to read certain journals on a regular basis, scanning for evidence around topics relevant to their practice. This activity needs to be planned into the working week.

Appraising evidence

Pharmacists should be competent to appraise the evidence in the following areas:

- a review article for:
  - a therapy
  - a test
  - health policy or management change.
- the quality of the following research methodologies:
  - systematic reviews
  - RCTs
  - qualitative research
  - case-control studies
  - surveys or cohort studies.
- the performance or outcome of an intervention against the following criteria:
  - acceptability
  - effectiveness
  - safety
  - patient satisfaction
  - appropriateness
  - quality
  - cost-effectiveness.

These appraisals must be conducted within the context of local circumstances that may affect the implementation of any research findings.

Storing and retrieving

If the above activities are in place then there is a clear need to ensure efficient storage and retrieval. This may consist of a tried-and-tested storage method, but ideally should include the ability to:

- enter references and abstracts using self-selected keywords into one of the personal bibliographic management systems
- search for references in that system
- download sets of references on to paper.

Drug information pharmacists should have the ability to cite references in their own reports by linking into the database.

References

1   Alarçon R de (1969) A personal medical reference index. *Lancet.* **1**: 301–5.

2   Haynes RB, McKibbon KA, Fitzgerald D *et al.* (1986) How to keep up with the medical literature: VI. How to store and retrieve articles worth keeping. *Ann Intern Med.* **105**. 978–84.

3   Sackett D, Haynes RB, Guyatt GH, Tugwell P (1991) *Clinical Epidemiology. A basic science for clinical medicine.* Little, Brown & Co., Boston/Toronto/London.

CHAPTER NINE

Generating knowledge

The place of pharmacy practice research (PPR)

Pharmacy is one of the most complex but least analysed healthcare services, according to the Pharmacy Practice R&D Task Force report.[1] In the current climate of change and demand for evidence, pharmacy finds itself without a research base that can underpin its development. Many developments have taken place but these have often been at a service level, with many different models. While there is general acceptance that change has been for the better and improvements have been cost-effective, supporting evidence is difficult to find.

Current status of PPR and how to develop it

It might be helpful to take hospital clinical pharmacy as an example. This development has grown steadily over the past 20 years and has developed into the practice of most hospital pharmacies in the UK. It is probably the most significant development in hospital pharmacy for many years. A review of research into hospital clinical pharmacy was published by Cotter and colleagues in 1995.[2] The authors' objective was 'To examine the evidence of the effectiveness or efficiency of clinical pharmacy service provision by UK NHS hospital pharmacies.'

The following types of study design were included in the review:

- prospective and retrospective

- before and after
- controlled and uncontrolled.

The search for relevant studies covered the following databases and methods:

- Medline from 1966 to 1994
- Embase from 1983 to 1994
- Pharmline from June 1978 to 1994
- International Pharmaceutical Abstracts from June 1970 to 1994
- manual search of journals and references in material identified
- personal communications with various researchers.

Evaluative studies for each service area were ranked according to three criteria: study strength, size of effect and generalisability, but there was no indication of how the inclusion criteria were applied, nor any assessment of the quality of studies or how data were extracted.

Table 9.1 shows the number and type of studies included in the review. This probably represents the majority of trials in this subject in the whole of the world literature, and reporting was only narrative.

The review reported the following results.

Table 9.1 Number of and type of studies included in review

Type of study	Number
Medication monitoring	6
Formation of hospital drug use policy	9
Provision of information	2
Provision of advice on therapeutics	6
Specialist services provided as part of a multidisciplinary team	8
Provision of educational services to healthcare personnel in secondary care	3
Provision of services directly to patients	16
Quality improvement studies	9
Specialist services	4
Provision of clinical pharmacy services to primary care recipients	1

- Pharmacists' recommendations to alter therapy were thought to improve the process of care but were rarely thought to have contributed significantly to patient care.
- The studies support, but not prove, the beneficial effects of pharmacist involvement in drug use policy in UK NHS hospitals. No study assessed the effects of drug policy on patient care or quality of life.
- No comprehensive evaluative studies have been carried out on drug information services.
- Two studies that are stronger in design indicate that pharmacists can have a moderate effect on the quality of prescribing and medication costs in geriatric medicine and psychiatry.
- Some studies provide weak evidence that pharmacist participation in team services improves the process of care, reduces drug expenditure and may improve patient outcome.
- There is little or no evaluative evidence on the role of hospital pharmacists in directly educating other pharmacists or health professionals in hospitals.
- No published studies evaluated the role of hospital pharmacists in research or clinical trials.
- Many studies of interventions that aimed to increase patients' knowledge of their therapy failed to measure changes in patients' medication-taking behaviour.
- Some studies suggest, but not prove, the effectiveness of pharmacy services in reporting adverse drug reactions.
- Central intravenous additives have not been properly evaluated. Few therapeutic drug monitoring service evaluations have been published.
- One study showed that savings can be made by hospital pharmacy involvement in the provision of medications to primary care, but it was not a full economic evaluation.

The authors concluded that few evaluations have been carried out on different categories of pharmacy services and, where they have, they have been limited in scope (concentrating mainly on short-term process and output variables), subject to potential bias and confounding, and have produced results that are not generalisable. No sound economic studies have been performed and studies on secondary outcome were very rare. Assessments of need were performed in some cases, but the aim seems to have been to show a need for a pharmacy service rather than to assess true need in an open-minded manner.

PPR attempts to understand the way in which pharmacy is practised and to evaluate the activities and interventions that pharmacists use to improve patient care. The task force mentioned above defined four strategic goals:

- to ensure that the research agenda addresses critical questions and healthcare priorities as well as the needs of the profession by establishing a mechanism to identify and prioritise the research agenda.
- to ensure that PPR is of an acceptably high standard by providing the support for practice-based researchers, establishing formal research networks, sponsoring training in research methods, and developing research leadership skills and enhanced career opportunities within both academic and practice environments.
- to foster an evaluative culture within pharmacy practice by encouraging all pharmacists to become 'research aware' from undergraduate level onwards and by encouraging wide publication and implementation of results.
- to ensure that PPR is adequately financed from both public and private sources and that the resources available for research are used to maximum effect.

These are high aims and some may be difficult to deliver. My four aims are given in Box 9.1.

Box 9.1   Four aims for pharmacy research

- To ensure that research is on the agenda of practising pharmacists both in hospital and community settings and that research skills are taught to undergraduates
- To find ways of encouraging and supporting pharmacy staff who want to carry out research
- To encourage all pharmacists to be aware of the importance of research and to find out what of all they do is supported by sound evidence
- To teach pharmacists how to compete for research funds

Review of pharmaceutical care research

A good illustration of the effects of this lack of underpinning research can be seen in a critical analysis of the pharmaceutical care research literature by Kennie et al.[3] Pharmacists have discussed pharmaceutical care since Hepler and Strand introduced the term in 1990.[4] Kennie et al. had four main objectives:

- to identify and describe studies that evaluate the provision of pharmaceutical care
- to critique the quality of research design and reporting
- to make recommendations aimed at improving the quality of pharmaceutical care research
- to create a reference for pharmaceutical care research conducted to the end of 1996.

What did they do?

They undertook a literature search of Medline and *International Pharmaceutical Abstracts* using the key phrase 'pharmaceutical care'. They also carried out a manual search of the Canadian journal *Pharmacy Practice*. Unfortunately, they did not search Embase, and the search they did was restricted to the English language, so is unlikely to be complete. The researchers then selected the relevant papers based on six criteria derived from the Strand definition of pharmaceutical care. Their criteria were:

- a pharmacist–patient relationship was established to involve the patient in drug therapy decisions
- desired outcomes were established in conjunction with the patient
- drug-related problems were identified
- drug therapy recommendations were made to the patient and/ or physician
- a method was indicated for monitoring and patient follow-up
- the pharmacists' activities were documented.

A 25-point instrument was developed; each criterion could score two points if present, one point if present and ill-defined and no points if not present.

What did they find?

Some 979 citations were identified and the number of publications per annum noted. This peaked in 1994. Of the 979 articles, only 57 were considered to potentially match the criteria and 43 of these were eliminated on closer examination. This left 12 articles for review with the following characteristics:

- setting of research: hospital, 6 studies; ambulatory care, 4 studies; community practice, 2 studies
- research design: case studies, 5; pre-post design, 3; clinical pharmacy versus pharmaceutical care, 1; randomised controlled trial, 3.

The scores made according to the check list were reported with a mean of 37 (range 31–46).

What recommendations did they make?

The authors made 15 recommendations under five different headings; these are summarised below.

- Pharmaceutical care terminology. The term 'pharmaceutical care' is often used when that use is not justified. Pharmaceutical care research is not clearly indexed in bibliographic databases. A disciplined approach is needed by researchers to differentiate pharmaceutical care from pharmacy services.
- Research design. There is an urgent need for good RCTs to assess the value of pharmaceutical care. Research reports must contain details of study subjects and the practice setting. There is also a need for standard data collection methods; the variety of data collected made any analysis difficult.
- Outcome measurements. The economic impact of pharmaceutical care should be evaluated alongside other outcomes.
- Standards. The authors argue that standards of pharmaceutical

care should be developed for the pharmacy profession. This seems to be optimistic, given that the term is used to cover a wide range of activities.

- Further research. It is not surprising that the authors call for more research, especially in the community pharmacy setting, and suggest that a pharmaceutical care research network be set up to co-ordinate activities and avoid duplication.

The clear message is that we need more research. There are plenty of people who are willing to provide opinions, but reliable evidence is the real need of the day.

Research in primary care pharmacy

This sector of pharmacy is perhaps the least well-served in terms of good evidence, and that which is available is rarely better than type IV or occasionally type III (*see* Table 2.1, p.15). What is available comes from a number of academic pharmacy practice units which have been established by pharmacy schools in the UK. This area is under considerable scrutiny by the UK Government as a potential source for delivering some of the new goals for improving primary healthcare; the danger is that we become driven by ideas and opinions rather than by quality evidence. One of the strengths claimed by community pharmacists is their ability to provide advice to consumers and patients. A recent research paper from Hassell and colleagues in Manchester sheds some light on this.[5]

The group observed the process of advice giving in ten pharmacies situated in a range of environments and with a wide range of dispensing workload. Observations were made over a period of one week (six days) and notes were taken. In addition, a sample of over 1000 customers were interviewed opportunistically. The group then classified the counsel given into one of five categories:

- product recommendation
- reassurance
- instruction
- information
- referral (e.g. to a medical practitioner).

Observed episodes ($n = 2379$) consisted of prescription-related requests (60%), non-prescription requests (29%) and response to symptoms and general health questions (5%).

What did consumers get?

- Advice giving, which was almost entirely product-based with little general advice.
- Didactic advice with emphasis on checking, instruction and information.
- Little in-depth dialogue about health and medicine needs.
- A concern about safety and potential interactions.

What did consumers want?

- Advice on effectiveness.
- To manage their own ailments.
- In practice, not very much.

The authors pointed out that the customers they interviewed were generally not happy with the concept of 'advice'. They see what pharmacy staff are doing as a form of helpfulness. The mismatch between consumer demand and perceived need (by the pharmacist) requires more work. The current discussion about making pharmacies the first port of call for health needs requires careful evaluation.

Developing research skills

Many pharmacists want to keep up to date, but many of the current methods have been shown not to work. The tried-and-tested methods of standard lectures, written information or learned texts, while remaining the backbone of many professional development programmes, just do not work.[6] Some of the time taken up by these programmes could be spent gaining research skills and undertaking simple, effective research based around the practice environment. There are a number of research skills courses available which provide basic research methodology with practical experience. It is far easier to learn alongside someone who is already involved in research, and such collaboration and co-operation can be very fruitful. Developing links with a local school of pharmacy can also lead to involvement in research.

Randomised controlled trials

Many of the research projects written up every year would have been far more informative had they been conducted as RCTs. The process of randomisation is not difficult, ethics committee approval is sometimes easier to obtain for this type of study and most patients do not object to being included in randomised studies, providing the reasons are explained to them.

Systematic review writing

Preparing systematic reviews is an important recognised research activity and is a task that has only just begun. In pain research, there are only 300 or so systematic reviews to date.[7] As with other forms of research, the skills are best learnt in collaboration with others and a team approach can probably help produce a sharper and more accurate review. The whole process of writing a review can give an appreciation of the work involved and of the importance of thoroughness in seeking to find the true answer to a question.

Joining the Cochrane Collaboration

The Cochrane Collaboration is built on the enthusiasm of individuals who collectively can make a difference. There are currently some 50 registered or proposed collaborative review groups covering virtually the whole of medicine. There is also a group looking at the evidence for effective professional practice. All these groups are open to receive new people willing to contribute something to the overall effort of producing maintaining and disseminating systematic reviews of evidence. This could be an offer to hand-search a journal you regularly receive or to be involved in a review. The collaboration is a supportive environment in which to develop new skills and sharpen old ones. Details of the review groups and of your nearest Cochrane Centre can be found in the *Cochrane Library*. Details of the main Cochrane Centres and Cochrane Websites are given in Appendix 3.

Developing a research culture

The element that is still missing within pharmacy practice is an obvious research culture. The incorporation of projects into postgraduate training courses, while producing some interesting though often unpublished material, has not helped to develop a research culture. This is probably due both to a mind-set that research is only linked to projects and to the pressures of service delivery. The medical model has overcome both of these by linking research activity to career progression is such a way that, for many clinicians, research activity becomes a way of life. This type of culture change needs to permeate pharmacy.

References

1   RPSGB (1997) *A New Age for Pharmacy Practice Research: promoting evidence-based practice in pharmacy*. Report of the Pharmacy Practice R & D Task Force.

2   Cotter SM, McKee M, Barber N (1995) *Hospital Clinical Pharmacy Research in the UK: a review and annotated bibliography*. Departmental Publication No.13. Dept of Public Health and Policy, London School of Hygiene and Tropical Medicine, London.

3   Kennie NR, Schuster BG, Einarson TR (1998) Critical analysis of the pharmaceutical care research literature. *Ann Pharmacotherapy*. **32**: 17–26.

4   Hepler CD, Strand LM (1990) Opportunities and responsibilities in pharmaceutical care. *Am J Hosp Pharm*. **47**(3): 533–43.

5   Hassell K, Noyce P, Rogers A, Harris J, Wilkinson J (1998) Advice provided in British community pharmacies: what people want and what they get. *J Health Serv Res Policy*. **3**(4): 219–25.

6   Sibley JC, Sackett DL, Neufeld VR (1982) A randomised trial of continuing medical education. *NEJM*. **302**: 511.

7   McQuay HJ *et al.* (1999) Systematic reviews in pain [Web page]. Available at www.jr2.ox.ac.uk/Bandolier/painres/MApain.html

CHAPTER TEN

Evidence for developing countries

Pharmaceutical services in developing countries face particular challenges that are significantly different from those faced by pharmacists in the so-called First World.

Medicines that are normally restricted to prescription in the UK may be readily available on general sale, while other extremely useful medicines such as morphine for severe pain may not be available at all or in such small quantities as to be effectively unobtainable. Many patients will not be able to afford all their prescribed medicines and so must choose which ones to buy. Doctors are supposed to make patients better, so often use irrational choices to achieve a cure. An example of this is prescribing several antibiotics for a single condition or prescribing injections where oral medication is sufficient. The quality of the medicines may be substandard or even dangerous. In the early 1990s, children in South Asia died as a result of consuming paracetamol elixir which contained ethylene glycol instead of propylene glycol. In addition, medicines may be poorly or inappropriately stored, thus rendering them useless at the time of sale or consumption.

Local pharmaceutical industry pressure, advertising and incentives may lead to irrational choices. Doctors can be offered large inducements to promote and prescribe certain medicines. On the other hand, patients may request the contraceptive agent that is advertised on the neon signs in the city centre or may believe that the famous brand name is bound to work better than a good-quality generic equivalent.

Ensuring medicines are available

Many developing nations have developed national drug policies, a concept that has been actively promoted by the WHO. For example, the national drug policy for Indonesia[1] drawn up in 1983 has the following objectives:

- To ensure the availability of drugs according to the needs of the population.
- To improve the distribution of drugs in order to make them accessible to the whole population.
- To ensure efficacy, safety quality and validity of marketed drugs and to promote proper, rational and efficient use.
- To protect the public from misuse and abuse.
- To develop the national pharmaceutical potential towards the achievements of self-reliance in drugs and in support of national economic growth.

To achieve these objectives, the following changes were implemented.

- A national list of essential drugs was established and implemented in all public sector institutions. The list is revised periodically.
- A ministerial decree in 1989 required that drugs in public sector institutions be prescribed generically and that pharmacy and therapeutics committees be established in all hospitals.
- District hospitals and health centres have to procure their drugs based on the essential drugs list.
- Most drugs are supplied by three government-owned companies.
- Training modules have been developed for drug management and rational drug use and these have been rolled out to relevant personnel.
- The central drug laboratory and provincial quality control laboratories have been strengthened.
- A major teaching hospital has developed a programme on rational drug use, developing a hospital formulary, guidelines for rational diagnosis and treatment guidelines for the rational use of antibiotics.

- Generic drugs have been made available at affordable costs to low-income groups.

Encouraging rational prescribing

One of the first challenges is to promote and develop rational prescribing, and a number of international initiatives exist in this area. WHO has actively promoted rational drug use as one of the major elements in its Drug Action Programme. In its publication *A Guide to Good Prescribing*[2] the process is outlined as:

- define the patient's problem
- specify the therapeutic objectives
- verify whether your personal treatment choice is suitable for this patient
- start the treatment
- give information, instructions and warnings
- monitor (stop) the treatment.

The emphasis is on developing a logical approach, and it allows for clinicians to develop personal choices in medicines (a personal formulary) which they may use regularly. The programme seeks to promote appraisal of evidence in terms of proven efficacy and safety from controlled clinical trial data, and adequate considera-tion of quality, cost and choice of competitor drugs by choosing the item that has been most thoroughly investigated, has favour-able pharmacokinetic properties and is reliably produced locally. The avoidance of combination drugs is also encouraged.

The routine and irrational use of injections should also be challenged. One study undertaken in Indonesia found that nearly 50% of infants and children and 75% of the patients aged five years or over visiting government health centres received one or more injections.[3] The highest use of injections was for skin disor-ders, musculoskeletal problems and nutritional deficiencies. Injec-tions, as well as being used inappropriately, are often administered by untrained personnel; these include drug sellers who have no understanding of clean or aseptic techniques.

Another group active in this area is the International Network for Rational Use of Drugs (INRUD, www.msh.org/dmp/inrud.html).

This organisation, established in 1989, exists to promote rational drug use in developing countries. As well as producing training programmes and publications, the group is undertaking research in a number of member countries, focused primarily on changing behaviour to improve drug use. One of the most useful publications from this group is entitled *Managing Drug Supply*.[4] It covers most of the drug supply processes and is built up from research and experience in many developing countries. There are a number of case studies described, many of which have general application for pharmacists working in developing countries.

In all the talk of rational drug use, the impact of the pharmaceutical industry cannot be ignored, with its many incentive schemes for doctors and chemist's-shop staff who dispense, advise or encourage use of particular products. These issues have been highlighted in a study of pharmaceutical sales representatives (medreps) in Bombay (Mumbai).[5] This was an observational study of medreps' interaction with pharmacies, covering a range of neighbourhoods containing a wide mix of social classes. It is estimated that there are approximately 5000 medreps in Bombay, roughly one for every four doctors in the city. Their salaries vary according to the employing organisation, with the multinationals paying the highest salaries. The majority work to performance-related incentives. One medrep stated 'There are a lot of companies, a lot of competition, a lot of pressure to sell, sell! Medicine in India is all about incentives; incentives to treat the patient well, incentives to doctors to buy your medicines, incentives for us to sell more medicines. Even the patient wants an incentive to buy from this shop or that shop. Everywhere there is a scheme, that's business, that's medicine in India.'

The whole system is geared to winning over confidence and getting results in terms of sales; this is often achieved by means of gifts or invitations to symposia to persuade doctors to prescribe. With the launch of new and expensive antibiotics worldwide, the pressure is to sell with little regard to the national essential drug lists or rational prescribing. One medrep noted that this was not a business for those overly concerned with morality. Such a statement is a sad reflection on parts of the pharmaceutical industry, which has an important role to play in the development of the health of a nation. It seems likely that short-term gains are made at the expense of increasing problems such as antibiotic resistance.

The only alternatives are to ensure practitioners have the skills to appraise medicine promotion activities or to more stringently control pharmaceutical promotional activities.

Rational dispensing

In situations where medicines are dispensed in small, screwed-up pieces of brown paper, the need for instructions to the patient takes on a whole new dimension. Medicines should always be issued in appropriate containers and labelled. While the patient may be unable to read, the next healthcare worker who seeks to help the patient is probably literate. There are many tried-and-tested methods in the literature for using pictures and diagrams to aid patient compliance. Symbols such as a rising or setting sun to depict time of day have also been used, particularly for treatments where regular medication is important, such as cases of tuberculosis or leprosy.[6]

Poverty may force patients to purchase one day's supply of medicines at a time, so it is important to ensure that antibiotics are used rationally and not just for one or two days' treatment. Often, poor patients need help from pharmacists to understand which are the most important medicines and to identify the prescribed items, typically vitamins, that can be missed in order to reduce the overall cost of the prescription to a more manageable level.

The essential drugs concept

The essential drugs list concept was developed from a report to the 28th World Health Assembly in 1975 as a scheme to extend the range of necessary drugs to populations who had poor access because of the existing supply structure. The plan was to develop essential drugs lists based on the local health needs of each country and to periodically update these with the advice of experts in public health, medicine, pharmacology, pharmacy and drug management. Resolution number 28.66 at the Assembly[7] requested the Director General to implement the proposal, which led subsequently to an initial model list of essential drugs (WHO Technical Series no 615, 1977). This model list has undergone regular review at approximately two-yearly intervals and the current 11th list was published in December 1999.[8] The model list is perceived by WHO to be an indication of a common core of medicines to cover most common needs. There is a strong emphasis on the need for national policy decisions and local ownership and implementation. In addition, a number of guiding principles for essential drug programmes have emerged.

- The initial essential drugs list should be seen as a starting point.
- Generic names should be used where possible, with a cross-index to proprietary names.
- Concise and accurate drug information should accompany the list.
- Quality, including drug content stability and bioavailability, should be regularly assessed for essential drug supplies.
- Decisions should be made about the level of expertise required for drugs. Some countries make all the drugs on the list available to teaching hospitals and have smaller lists for district hospitals and a very short list for health centres.
- Success depends on the efficient supply, storage and distribution at every point.
- Research is sometimes required to settle the choice of a particular product in the local situation.

The model list of essential drugs

The model list of essential drugs is divided into 27 main sections, which are listed in English in alphabetical order. Recommendations are for drugs and presentations. For example, paracetamol appears as tablets in strengths of 100 mg to 500 mg, suppositories 100 mg and syrup 125 mg/5 ml. Certain drugs are marked with an asterisk (previously a □), which denotes an example of a therapeutic group, and other drugs in the same group could serve as alternatives. The lists are drawn up by consensus and generally are sensible choices. There is currently an initiative under way to define the evidence that supports the list, and an example is shown in Table 10.1. This demonstrates the areas where RCTs or systematic reviews exist and serves to highlight areas either where further research is needed or where similar drugs may exist which have better supporting evidence.

Table 10.1 Evidence for analgesics named in the essential drugs list

Essential drug chapter	Drug	Systematic reviews	RCTs
1.2	Bupivacaine	+ (epidural)	+ +
1.2	Lignocaine	−	+ +
2.1	Aspirin	+	+ +
2.1	Allopurinol	− (in progress)	+ +
2.1	Indomethacin	−	+ +
2.1	Ibuprofen	+	+ +
2.1	Colchicine	−	+
2.2	Paracetamol	+ +	+ +
2.2	Codeine	−	− (as single agent)
2.2	Pethidine	−	+ +
7.2	Propranolol	−	+

In addition to work to strengthen the evidence base, there is a proposal to encourage the development of Cochrane reviews for drugs that do not have systematic review evidence.

Application of NNTs to the underpinning evidence should further strengthen the lists. At present, there is an assumption among doctors in some parts of the world that the essential drugs list is really for the poor of society and is somehow inferior. The use of NNTs around the analgesics in the list goes some way to disprove this and these developments may increase the importance of essential drugs lists.

Communicating clear messages

The impact of pharmaceutical representatives has already been discussed (Chapter 2) and the power of this approach has led to the concept of academic detailing to provide clear messages. A study by Thaver and Harpham[9] described the work of 25 private practitioners in an area around Karachi. The work was based on assessment of prescribing practices, and for each practitioner included 30 prescriptions for acute respiratory infections (ARI) or diarrhoea in children under 12 years of age. A total of 736 prescriptions were analysed and it was found that an average of four drugs were either prescribed or dispensed for each consultation. An antibiotic was prescribed in 66% of prescriptions, and 14% of prescriptions were for an injection. Antibiotics were requested for 81% of diarrhoea cases and 62% of ARI cases. Of the 177 prescriptions for diarrhoea, only 29% were for oral re-hydration solution. The researchers went on to convert this information into clear messages for academic detailing back to the doctors. Table 10.2 shows messages that emerged.

Table 10.2   Messages emerging from prescribing practices

Diagnosis	Message
Watery diarrhoea	'Watery diarrhoea needs water.' Give time to your patients, not antibiotics or antidiarrhoeals.
Cough and cold	More than 80% of upper respiratory infections are due to viruses and do not need antibiotics.
Cough and difficult breathing	'The wristwatch is more important than the stethoscope.' The diagnosis is pneumonia if the respiratory rate is high and chest widening is present.
Sore throat	'Take help from your friend the Penicillin.' WHO recommends penicillin in tonsillitis and related infections.
Diarrhoea treatment plan	'WHO-recommended plan for no, some and severe dehydration.' An easy-to-follow diagnosis and treatment protocol.
ARI treatment plan	'WHO-recommended plan for no, some and severe pneumonia.' An easy-to-follow diagnosis and treatment protocol.

The researchers went on to implement the programme and assessed the benefits. This was a nice piece of work based on developing messages that are supported by evidence.

Drug donations

It is a natural human reaction to want to help in whatever way possible when faced with human disaster, either as a result of some catastrophe or because of extreme poverty. Sympathetic individuals want to take action to help in a situation in which they would otherwise be helpless, and workers in difficult circumstances, only too aware of waste and excess at home, want to make use of otherwise worthless materials. The problem is that these situations do not lend themselves to objectivity. There are numerous accounts of tons of useless drugs being air-freighted into disaster areas. It then requires huge resources to sort out these charitable acts and often the drugs cannot be identified because the labels are not in a familiar language. In many cases, huge quantities have to be destroyed simply because the drugs are out of date, spoiled, unidentifiable or totally irrelevant to local needs. Generally, had the cost of the shipping been donated instead, then many more people would have benefited.

In response to this, WHO has generated guidelines for drug donations from a consensus of major international agencies involved in emergency relief. If these are followed, a significant improvement in terms of patient benefit and use of human resources will result.

Box 10.1 WHO guidelines for drug donations 1996

Selection of drugs
- Drugs should be based on expressed need, be relevant to disease pattern and be agreed with the recipient
- Medicines should be listed on the country's essential drugs list or WHO model list
- Formulations and presentations should be similar to those used in the recipient country

Quality assurance and shelf life
- Drugs should be from a reliable source and WHO certification for quality of pharmaceuticals should be used
- No returned drugs from patients should be used
- All drugs should have a shelf life of at least 12 months after arrival in the recipient country

Presentation, packing and labelling
- All drugs must be labelled in a language that is easily understood in the recipient country and contain details of

generic name, batch number, dosage form, strength, quality, name of manufacturer, storage conditions and expiry date
- Drugs should be presented in reasonable pack sizes (e.g. no sample or patient starter packs)
- Material should be sent according to international shipping regulations with detailed packing lists. Any storage conditions must be clearly stated on the containers, which should not weigh more than 50 kg. Drugs should not be mixed with other supplies

Information and management
- Recipients should be informed of all drug donations that are being considered or under way
- Declared value should be based on the wholesale price in the recipient country or on the wholesale world market price
- Cost of international and local transport, warehousing, etc, should be paid by the donor agency unless otherwise agreed with the recipient in advance

Evidence-based pharmacy practice

While modern practices, including the development of clinical pharmacy, are important, many basic issues await significant change in developing countries.

- Medicines can often be found stored together in pharmacological groups rather than in alphabetical order by type.
- Fridge space is often inadequate and refrigerators unreliable.
- There are different challenges, such as ensuring that termites don't consume the outer packages and labels or that storage is free of other vermin such as rats.
- Dispensary packaging and labelling can be woefully inadequate and patients leave with little or no understanding of how to take medicines which may have cost them at least one week's earnings.
- Medicines are often out of stock, not just for a few hours but for days or even weeks, particularly at the end of the financial year.
- Protocols and standard operating procedures are rarely found.

- Even when graduate pharmacists are employed, they often have little opportunity to perform above the level of salesperson, simply issuing medicines and collecting payment. For example, several hospital pharmacies in Mumbai, India, are open 24 hours per day for 365 days per year but only to function as retail outlets selling medicines to outpatients or to relatives of inpatients who then hand over the medicines to the nursing staff for administration.

Useful sources of information

A list of useful material about essential drugs programmes is available in Appendix 4.

Conclusions

Evidence is just as important in the developing world as it is in the developed world. Poverty comes in many forms and while the form we notice most is famine and poor housing, both of which are potent killers, medical and knowledge poverty are also significant. Evidence-based practice is one of the ways in which these problems can be minimised. Potentially, one of the greatest benefits of the Internet is the possibility of ending knowledge poverty and in turn influencing all the factors that undermine wellbeing. Essential drugs programmes have been a major step forward in ensuring that the maximum number benefit from effective drug therapy for disease.

References

1   World Health Organisation (1990) Review of the drug programme in Indonesia. Report of a WHO mission 16 October–3 November 1989. *DAP.* **90**(11): 1–36.

2   de Vries TPG, Henning RH, Hogerzeil HV, Fresle DA (1994) Guide to good prescribing. *WHO/DAP.* **11**: 1–108.

3   Management Sciences for Health (1988) *Health Centre Prescribing and Child Survival in East Java and West Kalimantan, Indonesia. Child survival pharmaceuti-*

cals in Indonesia, Part ii. Report of the Ministry of Health and Management Sciences for Health.

4   Management Sciences for Health (1997) *Managing Drug Supply: the selection, procurement, distribution, and use of pharmaceuticals.* Kumarian Press, Connecticut.

5   Kamat VR, Nichter M (1997) Monitoring product movement: an ethnographic study of the pharmaceutical sales representatives in Bombay, India. In: Bennett S, McPake B, Mills A (eds) *Private Health Providers in Developing Countries: serving the public interest?* Zed Books, London & New Jersey.

6   Georgiev GD, McDougall AC (1988) Blister calendar packs – potential for improvement in the supply and utilization of multiple drug therapy in leprosy control programs. *International Journal of Leprosy and Other Mycobacterial Diseases.* **56**(4): 603–10.

7   World Health Organisation (1985) *Handbook of Resolutions and Decisions of the World Health Assembly and Executive Board,* vol II 1973–1984. World Health Organisation, Geneva.

8   World Health Organisation (2000) Essential Drugs WHO Model List (revised 1999). www.who.int/medicines/edl/who_model_list_of_essential_drug.htm.

9   Thaver IH, Harpharm T (1997) Private practitioners in the slums of Karachi: professional development and innovative approaches for improving practice. In: Bennett S, McPake B, Mills A (eds) *Private Health Providers in Developing Countries: serving the public interest?* Zed Books, London & New Jersey.

Worldwide peer-reviewed journals in pharmacy

Extracted from *Ulrich's International Periodicals Directory* (38e) (2000). RR Bowker, New Providence, NJ. Published with permission.

Journal name	Contact address	Language and Internet site (where available)	Frequency of publication
Acta Pharmaceutica	Croatian Pharmaceutical Society, Masarykova 2, 10000 Zagreb, Croatia	English	Quarterly
Acta Pharmaceutica Turcica	ETAM AS, Matbaa Tesisleri, 26470 Eskisehir, Turkey	English, French or German, with summaries in Turkish www.anadolu. edu.tr	Quarterly

Journal name	Contact address	Language and Internet site (where available)	Frequency of publication
Acta Poloniae Pharmaceutica	Polskie Towarzystwo Farmaceut-yczne (Polish Pharmaceutical Society), UL Dluga 16, 00-238 Warsaw, Poland	English	Bi-monthly
Advanced Drug Delivery Reviews	Elsevier Science BV, PO Box 211, 1000 BM Amsterdam, Netherlands	English	Nine per year
Advances in Drug Research	Academic Press Inc, 525 B St, Ste 1900, San Diego, CA 92101-4495, USA	English	Irregular
Advances in Pharmaceutical Sciences	Academic Press Inc, 525 B St, Ste 1900, San Diego, CA 92101-4495, USA	English	Irregular
Advances in Pharmacology	Academic Press Inc, 525 B St, Ste 1900, San Diego, CA 92101-4495, USA	English	Irregular
Adverse Drug Reaction Bulletin	Wolters Kluwer NV, 227 E, Washington Sq, Philadelphia, PA 19106, USA	English and Italian www.lww.com	Bi-monthly

Journal name	Contact address	Language and Internet site (where available)	Frequency of publication
American Journal of Health System Pharmacy formerly *American Journal of Hospital Pharmacy*	American Society of Health System Pharmacists, 7272 Wisconsin Ave, Bethesda, MD 20814, USA	English www.ashp.org	Monthly
American Journal of Pharmaceutical Education	American Association of Colleges of Pharmacy, 1426 Prince St, Alexandria, VA 22314-2815, USA	English	Four per year
American Journal of Pharmacy	Philadelphia College of Pharmacy & Science, 600S 43rd St, Philadelphia, PA 19104-4495, USA	English	Quarterly
American Pharmaceutical Association Journal formerly *American Pharmacy*	American Pharmaceutical Association, 2215 Constitution Ave NW, Washington, DC 20037, USA	English	Bi-monthly

Journal name	Contact address	Language and Internet site (where available)	Frequency of publication
Annals of Pharmaco-therapy	Harvey Whitney Books Co, Box 42696, Cincinnati, OH 45242, USA	English www.theannals.com	Monthly
Apothecary	Healthcare Marketing Services, HCMS Inc, Box AP, Los Altos, CA 94023-2302, USA	English	Four per year
Australian Journal of Hospital Pharmacy	Society of Hospital Pharmacists of Australia, Level 11, 114 Albert Rd, South Melbourne, Victoria 3205, Australia	English www.shpa.org.au	Bi-monthly
Australian Pharmacist	Pharmaceutical Society of Australia, PO Box 21, Curtin, ACT 2605, Australia	English www.psa.org.au	11 per year
California Pharmacist	1112 I St, Ste 300, Sacramento, CA 95814, USA	English www.cpha.com	Quarterly
Californian Journal of Health System Pharmacy	725 30th St, Ste 208, Sacramento, CA 95816-3842, USA	English	Monthly

Journal name	Contact address	Language and Internet site (where available)	Frequency of publication
Canadian Journal of Hospital Pharmacy	Canadian Society of Hospital Pharmacists, 1145 Hunt Club Rd, Ste 350, Ottawa, Ontario K1V 0Y3, Canada	English and French	Bi-monthly
Canadian Pharmaceutical Journal	Canadian Pharmaceutical Association, 1785 Alta Vista Dr., Ottawa, Ontario ON K1G 3Y6, Canada	English	Ten per year
Ceska a Slovenska Farmacie	Czech Medical Association, Sokolska 31, 120 26 Prague 2, Czech Republic	Czech or Slovak with English summaries	Six per year
Clinical Drug Investigation	Adis International, Private Bag 65901, Mairangi Bay, Auckland 10, New Zealand	English	Monthly
Clinical Pharmaco-kinetics	Adis International, Private Bag 65901, Mairangi Bay, Auckland 10, New Zealand	English www.adis. com	Monthly

Journal name	Contact address	Language and Internet site (where available)	Frequency of publication
Drug Information Journal	Drug Information Association, 501 Office Center Drive, Ste 450, Fort Washington, PA 19034-3211, USA	English www. diahome.org	Quarterly
Drugs	Adis International, Private Bag 65901, Mairangi Bay, Auckland 10, New Zealand	English www.adis.com	Monthly
Drug Safety	Adis International, Private Bag 65901, Mairangi Bay, Auckland 10, New Zealand	English	Monthly
Drugs & Ageing	Adis International, Private Bag 65901, Mairangi Bay, Auckland 10, New Zealand	English	Monthly
Drugs & Therapy Perspective	Adis International, Private Bag 65901, Mairangi Bay, Auckland 10, New Zealand	English	Fortnightly

Journal name	Contact address	Language and Internet site (where available)	Frequency of publication
Eastern Pharmacist	507 Ashok Bhawan, 507 Nehru Place, New Delhi 110019, India	English	Monthly
EHP European Hospital Pharmacy	Medicultura International BV, C/o J Kotwas, Universitäts-klinikum, Steglitz Apotheke, Freie Universität Berlin, 12200 Berlin, Germany	English	Quarterly
European Journal of Pharmaceutical Sciences	Elsevier Science BV, PO Box 211, 1000 AE Amsterdam, Netherlands	English www.elsevier.com/locate/ejps	Six per year
Farmaceutski Glasnik	Croatian Pharmaceutical Society, Masarykova 2, 10000 Zagreb, Croatia	Croatia	Monthly
Farmacia Hospitalaria	General Orgaz 23, 1oA, 28020 Madrid, Spain	Spanish www.sefh.es	Bi-monthly
Farmacothera-peutica	Centro Brasileiro de Informacoes sobre Medicamentos, SCRN 712-713, Bloco G, No 30, 70760-770, Brasilia, Brazil	Spanish www.cff.org.br	Quarterly

Journal name	Contact address	Language and Internet site (where available)	Frequency of publication
Farmatsiya	PO Box 195, 10351 Moscow, Russia	Russian, with summaries in English	Bi-monthly
Formulary	Advanstar Communica- tions Inc, 7500 Old Oak Blvd, Cleveland, OH 44130, USA	English www.formulary journal.com	Monthly
Indian Journal of Hospital Pharmacy	Indian Hospital Pharmacy Association, R566 New Rajiner Nagar, New Delhi, 110060 India	English	Bi-monthly
Informazioni sui Farmaci	Via Doberdo 9, 42100 Reggio Emilia, Italy	Italian www.fcr.re.it	Bi-monthly
International Journal of Drug Policy	Elsevier Science BV, PO Box 211, 1000 AE Amsterdam, Netherlands	English www.elsevier. com/locate/ drugpo	Bi-monthly
International Journal of Pharmaceutics	Elsevier Science BV, PO Box 211, 1000 AE Amsterdam, Netherlands	English www.elsevier. com/locate/ ijpharm	38 per year
International Journal of Pharmacy Practice	Royal Pharmaceutical Society, 1 Lambeth High St, London SE1 7JN, UK	English	Quarterly

Journal name	Contact address	Language and Internet site (where available)	Frequency of publication
International Pharmacy Journal	FIP PO Box 84200, 2508 AE, The Hague, Netherlands	English, with summaries in French and Spanish www. pharmweb. net/ftp.html	Bi-monthly
Irish Pharmaceutical Journal	Irish Marine Press, 2 Le Glenageary Rd, Dun Laoghaire, Dublin 4, Ireland	English	Monthly
Journal of Chinese Pharmaceutical Sciences	Chinese Pharmaceutical Association, 38 Xueyuan Rd, Beijing 100083, People's Republic of China	English	Quarterly
Journal of Clinical Pharmacy & Therapeutics	Blackwell Scientific Publications Ltd, Osney Mead, Oxford OX2 OEL, UK	English www. blackwell-science.com	Bi-monthly
Journal of Euromed Pharmacy	University of Malta, Department of Pharmacy, Msida, Malta	English www.cis.um. edu.mt/~phcy/ euromed	Irregular

Journal name	Contact address	Language and Internet site (where available)	Frequency of publication
Journal of Geriatric Pharmacy	Haworth Press, Inc, 10 Alice St, Binghamton, NY 13904, USA	English	Quarterly
Journal of Oncology Pharmacy Practice	Stockton Press, C/o Nature America Inc, 345 Park Ave S, New York, NY 10010-1707, USA	English www. stockton-press. co.uk/jopp	Quarterly
Journal of Pharmaceutical Care in Pain and Symptom Control	Haworth Press, Inc, 10 Alice St, Binghamton, NY 13904, USA	English www.haworth pressinc.com	Quarterly
Journal of Pharmaceutical Medicine	Blackwell Scientific Publications Ltd, Osney Mead, Oxford OX2 0EL, UK	English	Quarterly
Journal of Pharmaceutical Sciences	American Pharmaceutical Association, 2215 Constitution Ave NW, Washington, DC 20037, USA	English Pubs.acs.org/ journals/ jpmsae/ index.html	Annual

Journal name	Contact address	Language and Internet site (where available)	Frequency of publication
Journal of Pharmaceutical Society of Korea	1489-3 Suhcho-3-dong, Sucho-gu, Seoul 137-073, South Korea	Korean, with English summaries	Bi-monthly
Journal of Pharmaco-epidemiology	Haworth Press, Inc, 10 Alice St, Binghamton, NY 13904, USA	English www.haworth pressinc.com	Quarterly
Journal of Pharmacy Teaching	Haworth Press, Inc, 10 Alice St, Binghamton, NY 13904, USA	English www.haworth pressinc.com	Quarterly
Journal of Pharmacy Technology	Harvey Whitney Books Co., Box 42696, Cincinnati, OH 45242, USA	English	Bi-monthly
Journal of Research in Pharmaceutical Economics	Haworth Press, Inc, 10 Alice St, Binghamton, NY 13904, USA	English www.haworth pressinc.com	Quarterly
Lyon Pharmaceutique	Secretaire Générale Hotel-Dieu de Lyon, 1 Place de l'Hôpital, 69288 Lyon Cedex 02, France	French www.univ-lyon1.fr/ispb/lyon-pharma	Eight per year

Journal name	Contact address	Language and Internet site (where available)	Frequency of publication
Michigan Pharmacist	Michigan Pharmacists Association, 815 N Washington Ave, Lansing, MI 48906, USA	English www.mipharm. com	Monthly
P & T (Pharmacy & Therapeutics)	Quadrant HealthCom, 26 Main St, Ste A, Chatham, NJ 07928-2402, USA	English	Monthly
Pakistan Journal of Pharmaceutical Sciences	University of Karachi, Faculty of Pharmacy, Karachi 75270, Pakistan	English	Two per year
Pharma Selecta	Stichting Pharma Selecta, Postbus 122, 8430 Oosterwolde, Netherlands	Dutch and English	Bi-weekly
Pharmaceutica Acta Helvetiae	Elsevier Science BV, PO Box 211, 1000 AE Amsterdam, Netherlands	English, French and German	Four per year
Pharmaceutisch Weekblad	Royal Netherlands Pharmaceutical Society, Alexanderstraat 11, 2514 The Hague, Netherlands	Dutch	Weekly

Journal name	Contact address	Language and Internet site (where available)	Frequency of publication
Pharmacists Letter	Therapeutic Research Centre, 2453 Grand Canal Blvd, Box 8190, Stockton, CA 95208, USA	English	Monthly
Pharmaco-economics	Adis International, Private Bag 65901, Mairangi Bay, Auckland 10, New Zealand	English	Monthly
Pharmaco-therapy	Pharmaco-therapy Publications Inc, New England Medical Center, Box 806, 750 Washington St, Boston, MA 02111, USA	English <u>www.iospress.nl</u>	Bi-monthly
Radiopharmacy & Radiopharma-cology	Gordon & Breach Harwood Academic, Poststrasse 22, 7000 Chur, Switzerland	English	Irregular
Real Academia de Farmacia Anales	Calle de Farmacia 11, 28004 Madrid, Spain	English, French and Spanish	Quarterly

Journal name	Contact address	Language and Internet site (where available)	Frequency of publication
Shengyang Yoake Daxue Xuebao	103 Wenhua Rd, Shenyang, Liaong 110015, People's Republic of China	Chinese	Quarterly
Therapeutic Drug Monitoring	Wolters Kluwer NV, 227 E Washington Sq, Philadelphia, PA 19106, USA	English www.lww.com	Bi-monthly
US Pharmacist	Jobson Publishing Inc, 100 Ave of the Americas, New York, NY 10013, USA	English www.uspharmacist.com	Monthly
Yaowu Fenxi Zazhi/ Journal of Pharmaceutical Analysis	Chinese Medical Association, Zhonghua Yixuehui, PO Box 2258, 42 Dongsi Xidajie, Beijing 100710, People's Republic of China	Chinese	Bi-monthly

Personal bibliographic software

Here are some of the products available. Most Websites allow downloads of a restricted package for evaluation.

EndNote 3.0
A complete package of search facility, reference organiser and bibliography creator. Available for Macintosh and PC, from Niles Software. Distributed in the UK by Cherwell Scientific Publishing, Oxford Science Park, Oxford OX4 4GA.
Web addresses: www.niles.com, www.cherwell.com

Idealist
Probably the most complex of those available. Details from Blackwell Science, Osney Mead, Oxford OX2 0EL (Tel +44 1865 206206).
Web address: www.blacksci.co.uk/products/idealist/aboutide.htm; however, the site only has contact details.

ProCite
Enables references to be gathered from a number of sources. Can be used to network or post databases on to the Web. Has a useful cite-while-you-write feature. Available for Macintosh and PC.
Web address: www.risinc.com

Reference Manager
Software to manage references from a variety of sources, including the Web. It is possible to network the databases and to create Web pages that enable access to databases. Available for PC only.
Web address: www.risinc.com

For both ProCite and Reference Manager contact Research
Information Systems, Brunel Science Park, Building 1, Brunel
University, Uxbridge UB8 3PQ. Web address: www.risinc.com
   A review of three of these products can be found on the Web at
www.biblio-tech.com/html/pbms.html

Contacts for the Cochrane Collaboration

Australasian Cochrane Centre
Mrs Kelly Binelli
Administrator
Australasian Cochrane Centre
Flinders Medical Centre
Bedford Park
South Australia
Australia 5042
Tel: + 61 8 8204 5399
Fax: + 61 8 8276 3305
Email: cochrane@flinders.edu.au

Brazilian Cochrane Centre
Dr Alvaro Nagib Atallah
Director
Centro Cochrane do Brasil
Universidade Federal de São Paulo – Escola Paulista de Medicina
Pedro de Toledo, 598
São Paulo
Brazil 04039-001
Tel: + 55 11 570 0469
Fax: + 55 11 575 6427
Email: cochrane.dmed@epm.br

Canadian Cochrane Network and Centre
Ms Judi Padunsky
Administrator
Canadian Cochrane Centre

c/o Health Information Research Unit
McMaster University Health Sciences Centre, Room 3H7
1200 Main Street
West Hamilton
Ontario
Canada L8N 3Z5
Tel: + 1 905 525 9140, ext 22520
Fax: + 1 905 546 0401
Email: jmorrisn@fhs.mcmaster.ca

Centre Cochrane Français
Ms Françoise Martin
Secretary CIT-CCF
Centre Léon Berard
28 Rue Laënnec
Lyon Cedex 8
France 69373
Tel: + 33 4 78 78 28 34
Fax: + 33 4 78 78 28 38
Email: fm@upcl.univ-lyon1.fr

Chinese Cochrane Centre
Prof Youping Li
Director
Chinese Cochrane Centre
The First University Hospital
West China University of Medical Services
Chengdu
Sichuan 610041
People's Republic of China
Email: cochrane@public.sc.cninfo.net

Dutch Cochrane Centre
Ms Marjan Loep
Administrator
Clinical Epidemiology and Biostatistics J2-221
Academic Medical Centre
Meibergdreef 15
PO Box 22700
Amsterdam
Netherlands 1100 DE
Tel: + 31 20 566 5602
Fax: + 31 20 691 2683
Email: cochrane@amc.uva.nl

German Cochrane Centre
Dr Gerd Antes
Institute for Medical Biometry and Medical Informatics
Hospital of the University of Freiburg
Stefan-Meier-Strasse 26
Freiburg i Br
Germany D-79104
Tel: +49 761 203 6715
Fax: +49 761 203 6712
Email: mail@cochrane.de

Italian Cochrane Centre
Dr Alessandro Liberati
Head of Department
Laboratory of Clinical Epidemiology
Mario Negri Institute
Via Eritrea 62
Milano
Italy 20157
Tel: +39 2 39014316
Fax: +39 2 33200231, +39-2-3560461
Email: cochrane@irfmn.mnegri.it

New England Cochrane Centre
Dr Joseph Lau MD
Co-Director
New England Cochrane Center
New England Medical Center
750 Washington Street Box #63
Boston
MA 02111
USA
Tel: +1 617 636 5133
Fax: +1 617 636 8032
Email: cochrane@es.nemc.org

Nordic Cochrane Centre
Dr Peter Gøtzsche MD, MSc
Director
Nordic Cochrane Centre
Rigshospitalet, Dept. 7112
Tagensvej 18 B
Copenhagen N
Denmark 2200

Tel: +45 3545 5571
Fax: +45 3545 7007
Email: general@cochrane.dk

San Antonio Cochrane Center
Cynthia Mulrow MD, MSc
Director
San Antonio VA Cochrane Center
Audie L Murphy Memorial Veterans Hospital
7400 Merton Minter Blvd (11C6)
San Antonio
TX 78284
USA
Tel: +1 210 617 5190
Fax: +1 210 617 5234
Email: cochrane@merece.uthscsa.edu

San Francisco Cochrane Center
Dr Lisa Bero and Dr Drummond
Rennie
Phillip Lollar, Administrator
San Francisco Cochrane Center
Institute for Health Policy Studies
1388 Sutter Street, 11th Floor
San Francisco
CA 94109
USA
Tel: +1 415 476 4958
Fax: +1 415 476 0705
Email: sfcc@sirius.com

South African Cochrane Centre
Dr Jimmy Volmink
Director
South African Cochrane Centre
Medical Research Council
19070 Tygerberg 7505
South Africa
Tel: +27 21 938 0911
Fax: +27 21 938 0310
Email: cochrane@eagle.mrc.ac.za

Spanish Cochrane Centre
Dr Xavier Bonfill MD, PhD
Director CEPSS
Spanish Cochrane Centre
Fundació Parc Taulí
Parc Taulí s/n
Sabadell (Barcelona)
Catalunya
Spain 08208
Tel: + 34 93 723 4094
Fax: + 34 93 723 3804
Email: cepss@siberia.chpt.es

UK Cochrane Centre
Ms Caroline Caldicott
Administrator
UK Cochrane Centre
Summertown Pavilion
Middle Way
Oxford OX2 7LG
UK
Tel: + 44 1865 516300
Fax: + 44 1865 516311
Email: general@cochrane.co.uk

Publications from the Department of Essential Drugs and Medicines Policy

* Indicates item is free of charge

General publications

*Essential Drugs Monitor
Periodical issued twice a year, covering drug policy, research, rational drug use and recent publications.

*WHO Action Programme on Essential Drugs in the South-East Asia Region
Report of an Intercountry Consultative Meeting, New Delhi, 4–8 March 1991. 49 pages, ref no SEA/Drugs/83 Rev.1.

National drug policy

*Report of the WHO Expert Committee on National Drug Policies
Contribution to updating the WHO Guidelines for Developing National Drug Policies. Geneva, 19–23 June 1995. 78 pages, ref no WHO/DAP/95.9.

Guidelines for Developing National Drug Policies
1988, 52 pages, ISBN 92 4 154230 6.

Indicators for Monitoring National Drug Policies
P Brudon-Jakobowicz, JD Rainhorn, MR Reich, 1994, 205 pages,
order no 1930066.

Selection and use

Rational Drug Use: consumer education and information
DA Fresle, 1996, 50 pages, ref no DAP/MAC/(8)96.6.

Estimating Drug Requirements: a practical manual
1988, 136 pages, ref no WHO/DAP/88.2.

The Use of Essential Drugs. Model list of essential drugs
Updated every two years. Currently 10th edition, 1999. The list is
available on the Internet at: www.who.int/medicines

Drugs Used in Sexually Transmitted Diseases and HIV Infection
1995, 97 pages, ISBN 92 4 140105 2.

Drugs Used in Parasitic Diseases (2e)
1995, 146 pages, ISBN 92 4 140104 4.

Drugs Used in Mycobacterial Diseases
1991, 40 pages, ISBN 92 4 140103 6.

Drugs Used in Anaesthesia
1989, 53 pages, ISBN 92 4 14101 X.

**Guidelines for Safe Disposal of Unwanted Pharmaceuticals In and
After Emergencies**
Ref no WHO/EDM/PAR/99.4.

Supply and marketing

*Guidelines for Drug Donations
Interagency guidelines, revised 1999. Ref no WHO/EDM/PAR/99.4.

*Operational Principles for Good Pharmaceutical Procurement
Essential Drugs and Medicines Policy / Interagency Pharmaceutical
Coordination Group, Geneva, 1999.

Managing Drug Supply (2e)
Management Sciences for Health in collaboration with WHO,
1997, 832 pages, ISBN 1-56549-047-9. Orders should be
addressed to Kumarian Press, 14 Oakwood Ave, West Hartford, CT
06119-2127, USA. Fax +1 860 233 6072. The cost is $84.95,
with a reduced cost of $22.95 for developing countries. Requests
for reduced-price copies should be sent to Kumarian Press using
institute or organisation letterhead.

Ethical Criteria for Medicinal Drug Promotion
1988, 16 pages, ISBN 92 4 154239 X.

Quality assurance

***WHO/UNICEF Study on the Stability of Drugs During
International Transport**
1991, 68 pages, ref no WHO/DAP/91.1.

Human resources and training

*The Role of the Pharmacist in the Health Care System
1994, 48 pages, ref no WHO/PHARM 94.569.

Guide to Good Prescribing
TPGM de Vries, RH Henning, HV Hogerzeil, DA Fresle, 1994, 108
pages, order no. 1930074. Free to developing countries.

Research

*No 1 Injection Practices Research
1992, 61 pages, ref no WHO/DAP/92.9.

*No 3 Operational Research on the Rational Use of Drugs
PKM Lunde, G Tognoni, G Tomson, 1992, 38 pages, ref no WHO/
DAP/92.4.

*No 24 Public Education in Rational Drug Use: a global survey
1997, 75 pages, ref no WHO/DAP/97.5.

*No 25 Comparative Analysis of National Drug Policies
Second Workshop, Geneva, 10–13 June 1996. 1997, 114 pages,
ref no WHO/DAP/97.6.

No 7 How to Investigate Drug Use in Health Facilities: selected drug use indicators
1993, 87 pages, order no 1930049.

How to order publications

For priced publications and a full list of WHO publications in the field of pharmaceuticals, contact: Marketing and Dissemination (MDI), World Health Organisation, 1211 Geneva 27, Switzerland. Fax: +41 22 791 4857; email: publications@who.ch

To obtain single copies of unpriced publications included in the list, contact: EDM Documentation Centre, Department of Essential Drugs and Policy, World Health Organisation, 1211 Geneva 27, Switzerland. Fax: +41 22 791 4167; email: edmdocentre@who. ch

Further information on EDM's publications and activities can also be found on the Internet at www.who.int/medicines

Useful Web addresses

- ACP-ASIM Journals and Information
  www.acponline.org/journals/journals.htm
- AHCPR Guidelines
  text.nlm.nih.gov/ then follow links
- American College of Clinical Pharmacy
  www.accp.com/
- American Society of Health System Pharmacists
  www.ashp.org/
- ARIF – Aggressive Research Intelligence Facility
  www.hsrc.org.uk/links/arif/arifhome.htm
- Australian Therapeutic Goods Administration
  www.health.gov.au/tga/
- *Bandolier*
  www.jr2.ox.ac.uk/Bandolier/
- Canadian Health Technology Assessment Programme
  www.ccohta.ca
- CASP – Critical Appraisal Skills Programme
  www.ihs.ox.ac.uk/casp/
- Center for Pharmaceutical Outcomes Research, North Carolina
  sunsite.unc.edu/pharmacy/Cepor/cepor.html
- Cochrane Collaboration
  hiru.mcmaster.ca/COCHRANE/DEFAULT.HTM
- Cochrane Library
  www.update-software.com/clibhome/clibdemo.htm
- Cochrane Pain, Palliative & Supportive Care
  www.jr2.ox.ac.uk/cochrane/
- Department of Health, UK: Research and Development
  www.open.gov.uk/doh/rdd1.htm
- DGV Homepage for European Union
  europa.eu.int/comm/dg05/index_en.htm
- Electronic Library – Journals & Newspapers
  www.santel.lu/SANTEL/DOCS/journals.html

- Equip – Essex-based GP magazine
  www.equip.ac.uk/
- EU Institutions
  europa.eu.int/inst-en.htm
- European Community Humanitarian Office
  europa.eu.int/comm/echo/en/
- European Society of Clinical Pharmacy
  www.escp.nl/data/welcome2.html
- GIDEON – Global Infectious Disease & Epidemiology
  www.cyinfo.com
- Guidelines Appraisal Project, McMaster, Canada
  hiru.mcmaster.ca/cpg/default.htm
- Health Services-Technology Assessment, USA
  text.nlm.nih.gov/
- IHS Library – filters for searching databases
  www.ihs.ox.ac.uk/library/filters.html
- International Federation of Pharmaceutical Manufacturers
  www.ifpma.org/
- International Network for the Rational Use of Drugs
  www.msh.org/dmp/inrud.html
- Management Sciences for Health
  www.msh.org/
- Medical Resources on the Internet
  planetree1.utmem.edu/NetResources/NetResources.html
- National Co-ordinating Centre for Health Technology Assessment
  www.soton.ac.uk/~wi/hta/
- National Pharmaceutical Association
  www.npa.co.uk/
- National Prescribing Centre
  www.npc.co.uk/
- NHS Centre for Reviews and Dissemination
  nhscrd.york.ac.uk/welcome.html
- NHS R&D Strategy, Anglia & Oxford
  wwwlib.jr2.ox.ac.uk/a-ordd/
- NIH Consensus Development Program, USA
  odp.od.nih.gov/consensus/
- Numbers needed to treat
  cebm.jr2.ox.ac.uk/docs/nnt.html
- Nursing & Health Care Resources on the Net
  www.shef.ac.uk/~nhcon/
- Oxford Centre for Evidence-Based Medicine
  cebm.jr2.ox.ac.uk
- Promoting Action on Clinical Effectiveness (PACE), King's Fund
  www.kingsfund.org.uk/pace/default.htm

- Pharm Info Net – interesting links pages
  pharminfo.com/phrmlink.html
- Pharmacy On-Line, Derby, UK
  www.priory.com/pharmol.htm
- Pharmacy Organisations via America Online
  users.aol.com/poison5249/GrierPharm/pharmorg.html
- Pharmaprojects
  www.pjbpub.co.uk/pharma/
- Royal Pharmaceutical Society of Great Britain
  www.rpsgb.org.uk/
- ScHARR: Netting the Evidence, School of Health and Related
  Research
  www.shef.ac.uk/~scharr/ir/netting.html
- Scottish Centre for Post Qualification Pharmaceutical Education
  www.strath.ac.uk/Departments/PharmSci/SCPPE.htm
- Scottish Intercollegiate Guidelines Network – SIGN
  pc47.cee.hw.ac.uk/sign/home.htm
- Sowerby Centre for Clinical Informatics
  www.schin.ncl.ac.uk/
- Turning Research into Practice (TRIP)
  www.gwent.nhs.gov.uk/trip/
- UK Medicines Control Agency
  www.open.gov.uk/mca/mcahome.htm
- UK Psychiatric Pharmacy Group – UKPPG
  www.ukppg.co.uk/
- Virtual Pharmacy Library, USA
  www.cpb.uokhsc.edu/pharmacy/pharmint.html
- Wessex DEC Service (Development and Evaluation Committee)
  www.soton.ac.uk/~dec/
- WHO Action Programme on Essential Drugs
  www.who.int/dap/
- WHO-OMS: World Health Organisation
  www.who.int/
- York Centre for Reviews and Dissemination
  www.york.ac.uk/inst/crd/sites.htm

Index

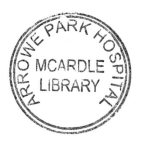